DENTISTRY WITHOUT MERCURY

by
Sam Ziff
Michael F. Ziff, D.D.S.

BIO-PROBE, INC.
ORLANDO, FLORIDA

Whenever a new discovery is reported to the scientific world, they say first, "It is probably not true."
Thereafter, when the truth of the new proposition has been demonstrated beyond question, they say, "Yes it may be true, but it is not important."
Finally, when sufficient time has elapsed to fully evidence its importance they say, "Yes, surely it is important, but it is no longer new."

Montaign
1533-1592

Four Hundred Years Later The Debate Over When Scientific Evidence Becomes "The Truth"
Continues Unabated!

Science is a hard taskmaster, and in the light of mounting evidence that suggestions of toxicity are for the most part ultimately confirmed by painstaking scientific inquiry, perhaps it is time to re-examine whether scientific standards of proof of causality--and waiting for the bodies to fall--ought not to give way to more preventive health policies that are satisfied by more realistic conventions and that lead to action sooner.
Editorial, New England Journal of Medicine (April 1987)

CONTENTS

DEDICATION

To that small group of dentists, other health care providers, and researchers whose primary motivation has been to bring the scientific facts about the potential dangers of silver/mercury dental fillings to the attention of their patients and the public. They have persisted in the face of overwhelming peer and establishment pressures and unmitigated harassment. They have suffered the indignities of being called quacks and frauds in national media publications and have continued to practice mercury-free because their motivating force has always been the health and well being of the patient.

Most of all this book is dedicated to those tens of millions of unsuspecting and trusting dental patients who have had the poison mercury implanted in their teeth, under the name of "silver dental fillings", without their knowledge and/or consent. This poison has the potential to seriously affect their health and will continually escape from the fillings and accumulate in their bodies as long as the poison remains implanted in their teeth.

INTRODUCTION

By
ALFRED V. ZAMM, M.D.

DENTAL MERCURY POISONING:
ONE OF THE FEW ECOLOGICAL POISONS
THE INDIVIDUAL CAN DO SOMETHING ABOUT

In my experience with many severely ill sensitive patients who exhibit allergic and other manifestations, removal of mercury ("silver"/"amalgam") dental fillings was the single most effective method of improving their health.

Air pollution, poisons in our food, toxins in our drinking water - all are ecological disasters reported on the front pages of our newspapers almost daily. Reporters often list catalogs of disastrous substances affecting our health - all beyond our control, all killing us every day on the installment plan, and all having a single common characteristic: something the individual can do nothing about. In contrast, the removal of dental mercury, a major toxin, is easily accessible to the individual, it is his own choice independent of society's behavior, and it is an act of preventive medicine that provides huge benefits at relatively minimal cost.

Should you take the poison out of your mouth? Should you not take this poison out of your mouth? Dentists are currently divided as to how to advise their patients.

Mercury ("silver") fillings are only 30 percent silver and 50 percent mercury. The choice of the appellation "silver" fillings obfuscates the fact that these "silver" fillings are actually 50 percent mercury. To call these fillings "silver" is not only inaccurate but is also misleading. The fillings should at least be named by that metal which is in the greatest concentration: mercury, and should be called for what they are: "mercury fillings." Another misleading term, "amalgam," is often used. The great majority of people do not realize that an amalgam is a solution of one or more metals in mercury. "Amalgam" is just another confusing term.

The consumer trying to make an educated choice is at a disadvantage from the very beginning because of these misleading terms. How many of us would have allowed poison fillings to be put into our mouths if they had been properly labeled as mercury fillings, and if the dentist had said "I am now going to put 50 percent mercury, a known poison substance into your mouth?"

Dentists are currently divided as to how to advise their patients; divided because in most cases the manifestations of the disease of mercury poisoning only starts to become apparent three to ten years after the insertion of the mercury.

The disease symptoms are insidious and overlap with the symptoms of many other diseases. Mercury poisoning is the greatest masquerader of our time. Dentists are not in a position to see the cause and effect relationship of the insertion of the mercury and the development of illness three to ten years later. Even the patient himself does not connect the illness to the original dental process. The "common complaints excerpt"(1), at the end of this introduction is particularly apt in elucidating the diversity of symptoms that occur in allergic disease, symptoms that the patient often does not connect to an allergic etiology. Many of these same symptoms are equally applicable to the symptoms of poisoning from mercury vapor.

It should be noted that there are many patients who have these identical symptoms who do not have either allergic disease or mercury poisoning; hence, these symptoms are not the exclusive domain of mercury poisoning or allergy; and, as mentioned above, there is much overlap. This is why the ability of mercury poisoning to masquerade is something one should be aware of. Furthermore, I have seen a number of patients who are edentulous, i.e., have no teeth and, hence, no mercury fillings, and who have had many of the symptoms in the above list. In a patient with mercury fillings it is impossible to predict a priori whether removal of the mercury fillings will reverse some of these symptoms. There are no prognostic tests. "Patch" tests are potentially dangerous because of the possibility of inducing allergic sensitivity in a patient who was not previously <u>allergic</u> to mercury but was <u>sensitive</u> to the toxic effect of mercury. We are talking about biological <u>sensitivity</u> to a poison - <u>not allergy</u> to a metal.(2)

One last note about predicting the outcome of mercury removal: the sickest patients I have seen are those with "mixed metals" in their mouths, i.e. gold and/or some other metal together with mercury fillings. They invariably do very well subsequent to the mercury removal.(3)

The evidence supporting these and similar observations is replete. Hundreds and hundreds of scientific references supporting these observations have been cited in the bibliographies of numerous books and the Bio-Probe Newsletters.(4-7)

The effectiveness and credibility of this point of view is evident. Every day more dentists declare their practices "mercury free," i.e., they will not insert mercury dental fillings. I predict that within five years the great majority of dentists will practice mercury-free dentistry. Perhaps the use of mercury will be declared illegal and the issue will be settled. Then professionals can go on to more productive activity than arguing about whether a poison is a poison.

Alfred V. Zamm, M.D. F.A.C.A., F.A.C.P.
111 Maiden Lane
Kingston, N.Y. 12401-4597

REFERENCES FOR DR. ALFRED V. ZAMM'S INTRODUCTION

1. Zamm A: Why Your House May Endanger Your Health. Simon & Schuster, New York, 1980. Touchstone Books, 1982.
2. Zamm, A: Letter to the editor. Bio-Probe Newsletter, 3(1):10-12, 1986.
3. Pleva, J: Mercury poisoning from dental amalgam. J Orthomol Psychiat. 12(3):184-193, 1983.
4. Ziff M.F., Hardy J.E., Goljan K., Vollmer D., and Wolf R.O. Bio-Probe Manual, 1984.
5. Ziff S. Silver Dental Fillings The Toxic Time Bomb. Aurora Press, New York, 1984.
6. Fasciana, G.S.: Are Your Dental Fillings Hurting You? Health Challenge Press, Springfield, MA 1986.
7. The Bio-Probe Newsletters. Volumes 1(1) to 8(1) incl. Orlando, FL, 1984-1991.

COMMON COMPLAINTS

that the sufferer may not attribute to a hypersensitivity to foods and/or inhalants.

ORGANS AND SYSTEMS PROBLEMS

1. Skin
   Rashes
   Excessive perspiration
2. Eyes
   Burning
   Itching
   Excessive tearing
   Feeling of heaviness and pressure
   within eyes
3. Ears
   Dizziness (Meniere's syndrome)
   Decreased hearing
   Buzzing in ears (tinnitus)
   "Plugged" ears
   (swollen eustachian tubes)
4. Nose
   Nasal obstruction
   Sinus congestion
   Sneezing (rubbing nose upward
   is a sign of allergy)
5. Throat
   Hoarseness
   "Itching" throat (leading to
   sore throat)
6. Lungs
   Excessive mucus
   Wheezing
7. Cardiovascular
   Palpitations
   Flushing
8. Gastrointestinal
   Nausea
   Loss of appetite
   Voracious appetite or sudden weight gain
   (5 pounds in 2 days)
   Chronic obesity
   Excessive thirst
9. Genitourinary
   Urgent urination
   Frequent urination
   Bedwetting
   Vaginal itching
   Excessively painful menstruation
10. Muscular-skeletal
    Muscle soreness
    Joint pains
    Uncertain gait

GENERAL PHYSICAL PROBLEMS

1. Fatigue (physical or mental)
2. Loss of former energy ("getting old")
3. Weakness
4. Edema (swelling)
5. Pallor
6. Inappropriate chilliness or
   excessive warmth
7. Excessive perspiration without fever
8. Unexplained fevers

NERVE AND MUSCLE PROBLEMS

1. Fainting
2. Blurred vision
3. Unexplained hyperactivity
4. Headache
5. Dizziness

MOOD CHANGES

1. Unexplained anxiety
2. Unwarranted excitability
3. Unexplained irritability
4. Hostility
5. Aggression
6. Insomnia
7. Restlessness
8. Difficulty concentrating
9. Difficult thinking
10. Mental confusion
11. Grogginess
12. Decreased reading comprehension
13. Forgetfulness
14. Difficulty recalling words
15. Depression
16. Loss of interest in work or former
    activities or hobbies
17. Crying spells
18. Tendency for fixed ideas; recycling
    or repeating of ideas
19. Antisocial behavior
20. Thoughts of suicide

8

QUESTIONS AND ANSWERS ABOUT SILVER AMALGAM FILLINGS

WHAT IS SILVER AMALGAM?

Silver amalgam, commonly referred to as "silver fillings," is the material most often used by dentists to fill the cavities caused by tooth decay. The term "amalgam" is a type of metal alloy (mixture) which contains mercury, a poison more toxic than lead or arsenic.. Silver amalgam, developed by a British chemist in 1819, was originally made by filing down silver coins and mixing the filings with some mercury to make a paste or pliable mass. Today modern amalgam also contains copper, tin and zinc. Many of the newer amalgams have fairly high levels of copper, also known to have toxic properties. The problem with calling this dental material silver amalgam is that it does not make obvious the fact that the major component is mercury. This material should really be called "mercury fillings." In fact, most people, including a great number of physicians, are not aware that all those "silver fillings" in their mouths each contain up to 50 percent mercury. If they did, they may choose not to have it placed in their teeth.

Why has this mercury filling material been used for over 150 years by dentists? The pliable mass containing mercury, silver and other metals undergoes a chemical reaction causing the material to harden after it has been placed into a cavity. This was quite an innovation for the dental profession. It allowed greater numbers of people to be treated at less cost, since before the discovery of mercury fillings the only options available were gold fillings or tooth extraction. Consequently, mercury fillings catapulted dentistry from a cottage industry serving only the wealthy enough to afford it, to the health industry of today serving hundreds of millions of the world population.(1).

ARE THE MERCURY FILLING MATERIALS SAFE?

There is no simple answer to this question. In fact, it has been asked repeatedly for over 150 years of mercury use in dentistry.

Mercury is a known poison. It is also very volatile. This means that "metallic" mercury gives off mercury vapor when agitated, compressed or exposed to increases in temperature. Mercury vapor - which is colorless, tasteless and odorless - if inhaled into the lungs can pass into your blood stream for distribution to all body tissues. Dentists have always been taught to believe that once mercury has been combined into the filling material, it remains "locked in" and can't come out.

In fact, as late as January 1984, the American Dental Association (ADA) was publishing information that stated "When mercury is combined with the metals used in dental amalgam, its toxic properties are made harmless."(2) In 1985 that statement was changed to "...Mercury is made virtually harmless when it combines with the other metals used to produce amalgam."(3) In 1991, the statement was again changed and now reads "...It is important to note that mercury forms a biologically inactive substance when it combines with the other materials used to produce amalgam."(4) The sad fact is that no scientific evidence exists to support any of the statements. In fact, and quite to the contrary, scientific data clearly demonstrates that dental amalgam is an unstable product.(5) The ADA is evidently completely aware of this fact because their document on the handling of mixed scrap amalgam (the portion not used in completing the filling) states that it must be stored in an air tight container under X-ray fixer and disposed of as hazardous waste.(6)

Until recently, most dentists believed what they were taught in school and what the ADA had to say about mercury staying "locked in." Now, however, there is scientific evidence proving that the mercury does not stay locked in and that its toxic properties are not made harmless. Scientific evidence from the University of Iowa, University of Calgary, Oral Roberts University and New Zealand clearly shows that mercury vapor escapes from the amalgam fillings in your teeth.(7-11)

Confirmation of the escape of mercury vapor and ions from amalgam dental fillings is provided by The World Health Organization (WHO) Environmental Health Criteria 118 document (EHC 118) on inorganic mercury. The WHO document clearly states that the largest estimated average daily intake and retention of mercury and mercury compounds in the general population, not occupationally exposed, is from dental amalgams, not from food or air. The estimated average daily intake of mercury from dental amalgams being 3.8-21 micrograms per day.(12)

Table 2 on page 36 of the WHO Health Criteria 118 document displays the following information:

Table 2. Estimated average daily intake and retention (ug/day) of total mercury and mercury compounds in the general population not occupationally exposed to mercury[a]

Exposure	Elemental mercury vapour	Inorganic mercury compounds	Methylmercury
Air	0.030 (0.024)	0.002 (0.001)	0.008 (0.0064)
Food			
Fish	0	0.600 (0.042)	2.4 (2.3)
Non-fish	0	3.6 (0.25)	0
Drinking-water	0	0.050 (0.0035)	0
Dental amalgams	3.8-21 (3-17)	0	0
Total	3.9-21 (3.1-17)	4.3 (0.3)	2.41 (2.31)

[a] From: Environmental Health Criteria 101: Methylmercury (WHO 1990)

Values given are the estimated average daily intake; the figures in parentheses represent the estimated amount retained in the body of an adult.

Values are quoted to 2 significant figures.

More startling than the WHO conclusions was a recent 1992 study done by Professor Aposhian and his colleagues at the University of Arizona demonstrating that two-thirds of the body burden of mercury of those with dental amalgams appears to be derived originally from the mercury vapor released from their amalgams.(13) A similar study completed

11

in Germany by Zander and his colleagues provided data demonstrating that the release of mercury from amalgam fillings represents the main source of mercury exposure in subjects with amalgam fillings.(14) The significance of the data from these studies is that the daily dose exposure required to give that large a tissue concentration, is much greater than any previously shown by intra-oral or exhaled mercury vapor data. Consequently, rather than the overestimation of intra-oral vapor the pro-amalgam "experts" would have everyone believe, it now appears that most of the published scientific studies have grossly underestimated the actual amount of mercury released from amalgam dental fillings.

WHAT CAUSES THE MERCURY TO ESCAPE?

That is an interesting question, for which science is continually producing new data and answers. For example, very little scientific significance was previously given to the unstimulated release of mercury from amalgam fillings. All of the attention was focused on the amount of mercury vapor released during actual stimulation by chewing. However, recent research in Sweden has concluded that the static unstimulated release of mercury vapor from amalgam fillings, which goes on 24 hours a day 365 days a year, is a major contributor to total mercury body burden.(15)

More recently, a 1992 study by Professor Skare of Sweden found that fecal excretions of mercury were twenty times greater than the corresponding urinary excretion. Moreover, amalgam bearers with a large number of fillings showed a fecal excretion of total-mercury that was 100 times larger than the mean intake of total-mercury from a normal Swedish dietary intake (2 mcg Hg/24 hour). Individuals, loaded with an average number of amalgams, are predicted to show a fecal total-mercury excretion of 60 mcg Hg 24/hours, thus exceeding the existing WHO-standard concerning the maximum allowable intake of total-mercury from food of 45 mcg Hg/24 hours.(16-17)

Successive scientific research has now demonstrated: 1) large amounts of mercury vapor being released during chewing and continuing for an additional 90 minutes after stimulation; 2) static unstimulated release of mercury vapor goes on continuously 24 hours a day; and 3) confirmation of studies done by Stock in 1934 and Frykholm in 1957 demonstrating that the body uptake from inorganic mercury swallowed with saliva can be as much as hundreds of micrograms per day for individuals with a large number of amalgam fillings.(18-19)

Whether stimulated release is caused by the grinding and chewing action, or an increase in temperature, really doesn't matter. The important point to remember is that mercury vapor and abraded ion particles are escaping and being inhaled and swallowed as well as being absorbed by the oral and nasal mucosa continuously during the lifetime of an amalgam filling.(20)

There is also another phenomenon that occurs in the mouth that can contribute to the release of mercury and it is called corrosion. Corrosion is similar to "rust" and means that surface particles of the filling material are being chemically broken down and released into the oral cavity. Mercury vapor is released when you chew or grind and, in addition, minute rusted particles of the amalgam are being abraded and taken up by your food or saliva and swallowed. These minute particles of mercury filling may be acted upon by intestinal enzymes and bacteria to produce methylmercury, an even more toxic form than elemental mercury. However, the significance of this effect has not been fully determined. Much more significant than the potential to produce methylmercury is the discovery that mercury from amalgam dental fillings causes gingival and intestinal microflora to become mercury resistant and antibiotic resistant.(21) The fact that so many people have become antibiotic resistant is something that has baffled and deeply concerned the medical profession because it is creating so many serious problems in the successful treatment of infectious diseases.

WHAT CAUSES THE CORROSION (RUSTING)?

Amalgam, like most other metals, when exposed to moisture and oxygen will rust or oxidize. A car battery has two or more dissimilar metals suspended in an acid solution. The corrosion that results produces free electrical currents. In your mouth, the amalgam fillings (normally having 4 or 5 different metals) provide the dissimilar metals and your saliva provides the electrolyte (saliva contains various elements such as calcium, magnesium, potassium and acid). So, you have all the ingredients available in your mouth to create electrical currents. Indeed, these electrical currents can be measured. This phenomenon is called "oral galvanism" and literally means that your oral cavity is like a small car battery or miniature electrical generator. When your miniature battery starts generating electrical current, the process of corroding (i.e. break down) of amalgam fillings is increased. This increases both the amount of mercury vapor and abraded particles that can be released into the oral cavity.(22) It can also be instrumental in the release of free-mercury droplets from the filling.(23)

CAN ORAL GALVANISM CAUSE OTHER PROBLEMS?

Yes. Although just saying "yes" is an oversimplification. There is scientific evidence that in addition to amplifying the corrosion problem, some individuals are very susceptible to these internal electrical currents. It is a very complex problem and scientists still don't have all the answers. For instance, it is not really known whether the electrical currents themselves cause problems or whether the problems are being caused by the electrical currents forcing metal ions from mercury fillings into the cells and bones of the oral cavity, or causing their transport into the brain via the trigeminal nerves or valveless venous pathways. There are a multitude of case histories that could be used to defend any of the arguments. From your standpoint as a patient, the important thing to know is that dissimilar metals in the mouth can contribute to electrical activity and corrosion and that in some individuals this can cause unexplained pain, ulcerations, inflammation, etc.(24)

Another aspect of this overall problem is that electrolytic corrosion can be enhanced by gold and mercury fillings being in contact. So, if there is a mercury filling under a gold in contact. So, if there is a mercury filling under a gold crown or if a gold filling or crown is in contact with an opposing or adjacent amalgam filling, it could exacerbate corrosion and increase the release of mercury particles and vapor into the oral cavity. Even standard dental textbooks have warned against this for years.(25)

WHAT IS THE AMERICAN DENTAL ASSOCIATION'S (ADA) POSITION ON THE RELEASE OF MERCURY FROM AMALGAM FILLINGS AND ITS POTENTIAL TO HARM HUMANS?

In July of 1984, the National Institute of Dental Research (NIDR) sponsored and the ADA hosted a "Workshop On The Biocompatibility of Metals In Dentistry." After this workshop, the ADA officially acknowledged that mercury is released from amalgam fillings. However, they went on to state that the amount released is so small that it could not cause any health problems except in those individuals who might be hypersensitive or allergic to mercury.(26) That position has remained essentially unchanged. In fact, in the December 1987 issue of the Journal of the American Dental Association (JADA), the ADA went to great lengths to publish a review article of the scientific literature that ended with a conclusion to support their official policy, i.e.:

"Occupational exposure to mercury is a potential hazard for dental personnel, but is completely preventable with the implementation of proper mercury hygiene practices. There is no evidence in the scientific literature that the minute amounts of mercury vapor that may be released from amalgam restorations cause mercury poisoning. Allergic reactions to mercury and other constituents of amalgam have been documented, but are exceedingly rare. The association between allergies and oral lichen planus requires further investigation. Finally, dental amalgam, which has been used extensively for more than 100 years, has an exemplary record of safety and benefit to the dental patient."

There are several problems with the ADA position:

1. To a large extent, the ADA position on the release and potential toxicity of mercury vapor from amalgam dental fillings is based on exposure, urine mercury, and health studies of chlor-alkali workers. These workers were all simultaneously being exposed to both chlorine gas and mercury vapor, which is certainly not the case with dental staff and individual amalgam bearers.

Chlorine gas reacts spontaneously with elemental mercury vapor in air.(27) As early as 1904 scientists were aware of this reaction and determined the best way of protecting workers in mirror factories was to induce and maintain a low chlorine content in the air (Mercury was used in the creation of the black reflecting surface applied to the back of the glass).(28) When elemental mercury is exposed to the chlorine gas, it is then oxidized to the much less toxic mercurous chloride (calomel).(29)

Italian researchers found precipitated calomel in mercury-using chlorine factories. They also studied rats exposed only to mercury vapor and compared the animals to others exposed to a mixture of chlorine and mercury. Exposure to the mixture in the same proportions as in the chlorine factories but at higher levels, was strikingly less toxic than exposure to mercury vapor alone. Experimental animals exposed only to mercury suffered severe neurological symptoms while those exposed to the mixture of mercury and chlorine displayed only mild gastrointestinal disorders. The difference in symptomatology can be explained by the fact that the brains and hearts of the rats exposed to the mixture of mercury and chlorine had only 8-10% of the mercury levels found in the rats exposed to mercury only.(27-29)

2. Certain scientific articles, very damaging to their position, were omitted in their review of the literature. Two of these, Djerassi and Berova (1969) and Miller et al. (1987), demonstrate clearly that the percentage of allergy to amalgam and/or mercury can be as high as 44.3%.(30-31) That percentage, of course, would not permit the ADA to make the statement "Allergic reactions to mercury and other

constituents of amalgam have been documented, but are exceedingly rare."

3. Additionally, none of the ADA statements, apparently designed to lull the dental profession and the American people into a false sense of security regarding the continued use of amalgam, can be substantiated scientifically. In a recent position paper in the Journal of the American Dental Association (April, 1990), the current adjusted ADA position on the safety of dental amalgam is reconciled as:

> "The strongest and most convincing support we have for the safety of dental amalgam is the fact that each year more than 100 million amalgam fillings are placed in the United States. And since amalgam has been used for more than 150 years, literally billions of amalgam fillings have been successfully used to restore decayed teeth."(32)

Think about that! The ADA is providing the worst kind of "anecdotal" evidence as their scientific proof that amalgam fillings are safe. What they are really saying is THAT THEY HAVE ABSOLUTELY NO SCIENTIFIC EVIDENCE PROVING THAT THE MERCURY RELEASED FROM AMALGAM FILLINGS IS NOT CAUSING MERCURY POISONING.

The ADA must be terribly concerned about the tenuous legal nature of their position on the safety of amalgam. Otherwise, there couldn't be any rational reason for their recent action revising their Principles of Ethics and Code of Professional Conduct, Section 1-J, making it improper and unethical to remove amalgam restorations from the non-allergic patient for the alleged purpose of removing toxic substances from the body, when such treatment is performed solely at the recommendation or suggestion of the dentist.

We feel quite strongly that such action violates the constitutional rights of the dentist to advise his patient of the potential dangers of mercury and your rights as a patient to have a freedom of choice in the matter of dental materials to be placed in your mouth. It is apparent that the ADA is worried about their previous statements because they are spending a great deal of money lobbying to defeat "Informed Consent" legislation in Illinois, Colorado, New Mexico, and California. Their message to the Legislators is quite simple, i.e., amalgam is safe, so why do you need the patient's consent? You only get an informed consent signed when there is a potential risk! Fortunately, they were not totally successful in California. California did pass into law legislation requiring that the Board of Dental Examiners of California develop and distribute a fact sheet describing and comparing the risks and efficacy of the various types of dental restorative materials in the treatment of dental patients. The data sheets are to be available in every dental office.

You should be aware that in the more than 125 years that the ADA has been in existence, it has not funded one single research project proving the biocompatibility or safety of dental amalgam in humans. The same can be said for the NIDR during the term of its existence as the dental research arm of the National Institutes of Health (A U.S. Government Agency), even though one of their primary responsibilities is to fund dental research investigating the biocompatibility of dental materials. This means that for 150 years the dental profession has been placing mercury/amalgam fillings in patients without ever determining its safety.

Conversely, on the other side of the amalgam safety question, there has been a proliferation of hard scientific evidence clearly demonstrating very serious questions of safety and attendant ethical considerations concerning further implantation of the poison mercury in humans.

There is conclusive scientific research showing a direct correlation between the numbers and surfaces of amalgam fillings and the mercury content of brain tissue.(33-35) As science in all of its research on mercury (over 12,000 scientific studies,(36)) has not been able to determine one single human requirement for this poison, a rational person must ask of what benefit this accumulation of mercury in their brain could be? Conversely, could it be detrimental or even hazardous? Certainly, the ADA has no scientific proof that it isn't causing damage. They can't, for example, say with any scientific authority that it isn't a contributing factor in emotional disorders or Alzheimer's disease.

Quite the opposite appears to be true. Over the past several years, teams of medical researchers at the Sanders Brown Center For Aging at the University of Kentucky (UK) have been investigating Alzheimer's disease (AD). Autopsy studies of the brains of Kentuckians who died from AD have demonstrated "strikingly" high levels of mercury. This presented the very puzzling question of how could these individuals, from all over the state of Kentucky, having no occupational exposure to mercury, all have high levels of mercury in their brains? In an effort to answer that question, the UK has recently received a $760,000.00 grant to investigate whether a causal relationship exists between amalgam dental fillings and the development of Alzheimer's disease.(37-39)

One of the most disturbing aspects of the ADA position on the replacement of amalgams is that some of the foremost research toxicologists have recently concluded "The release of mercury from dental amalgams makes the predominant contribution to human exposure to inorganic mercury including mercury vapor in the general population."(12, 40) Admittedly, these researchers have not said that the mercury being released is causing any damage. However, they have not said it isn't and they have not said that mercury is not a poison and they have not said that mercury being released from amalgam fillings is good for us. They have, however, stated that no amount of exposure to mercury vapor can be considered harmless. So, it would appear that the ADA, through amendment of its Code of Ethics, wants to insure that you continue to increase your body burden of mercury in the brain, pituitary, hypothalamus, thyroid, heart, lungs, liver, kidneys, etc. and in pregnant women, the tissues in your unborn babies.

WHAT ARE THE FDA RESPONSIBILITIES ON MIXED AMALGAM?

By law, the Food and Drug Administration (FDA) is required to classify all medical (including dental) devices accepted for use in the United States. If a material is not classified under the law it cannot be considered an approved dental device. The Final Rule of the FDA on Classifications of Dental Devices was published in the Federal Register on 12 August 1987. There is no mention or classification of dental amalgam as a dental device. What was approved and classified were the components of amalgam: Mercury was placed in Class I and amalgam alloy (what is mixed with the mercury to form amalgam) was placed in Class II. Interestingly, neither component by itself can be used as a dental device, which is also not in accordance with the law as it requires each dental device to be safe and effective. If it can't be used by itself to fill a cavity, how can it be effective and an approved dental device?

The rationale behind not classifying dental amalgam was that it is a "reaction product" prepared in the dental office. This is a clear violation of the intent of Congress and The Medical Device Amendment to the Federal Food, Drug, and Cosmetic Act signed into law on 28 May 1976. In essence, this was a maneuver to circumvent the need to identify dental amalgam as an implant. The FDA definition of an implant is "Implant means a device that is placed into a surgically or naturally formed cavity of the human body. A device is regarded an implant for the purpose of this part only if it is intended to remain implanted continuously for a period of 30 days or more, unless the commissioner determines otherwise in order to protect human health."(FR 43 32994, July 29, 1978) Implants must be placed in Class III, requiring scientific proof of safety. This definition was reaffirmed by the Safe Medical Devices Act of 1990. (PL 101-629)

The argument that it is a "reaction product" mixed in the dental office is specious. The amalgam manufacturer provides both components of dental amalgam in a single capsule, separated by a membrane. The amalgam manufacturer also determines how much mercury is placed in the capsule and the metallic content (formula) of the dental alloy placed in the capsule. All the dentist or his staff can do is follow the exact instructions of the manufacturer in placing the capsule in a machine that mixes the two components together producing the "reaction" product that is finally implanted in a living tooth. The dental staff has absolutely no control over determining the content of the mixed amalgam. It is patently clear that the FDA should have classified dental amalgam in Class III and demanded that the amalgam manufacturer provide proof of the safety of the mixed amalgam implant. The Commissioner of the FDA should place an immediate moratorium on further use of dental amalgam until it has been proven safe to implant in humans.

However, it does not appear that any such action will be taken. Instead, an effort is being made to circumvent the need to determine the safety of mixed amalgam and to classify it by proposing to call mercury and the amalgam alloy a kit. The kit would have the highest classification of any of its components which would be the class II category of the amalgam alloy.(41) Classifying it as a kit will avoid the need to determine the safety of the mixed "reaction" product that is finally implanted in the teeth of humans.

WHAT ARE THE POTENTIAL HEALTH PROBLEMS THAT COULD BE CAUSED BY MERCURY VAPOR ESCAPING FROM AMALGAM FILLINGS?

Now that it has been conclusively proven and documented that the mercury is not "locked into" dental amalgam, researchers have begun to trace its body accumulation and effects. Since the established dental community has elected to avoid the subject, medical scientists have joined the few interested dentists in conducting the investigations. Basically, the issue has now passed out of the domain of the dental profession into the hands of the medical and scientific communities.

A research team at the University of Calgary School of Medicine initially published two animal studies tracing dental amalgam mercury into the tissues of sheep. In the latter study the distribution of dental mercury was also traced into the tissues of pregnant ewes and their unborn babies. The team includes M.D. and Ph.D. medical scientists and one dentist, Murray J. Vimy, D.M.D.(42-43)

Utilizing radioactively labelled mercury to prevent mistaken identification of mercury from other sources, amalgam fillings were placed in the chewing surfaces of molar teeth and traced into body tissues. In a second study the same technique was used on pregnant sheep. Within two days, the amalgam-derived mercury was found in the maternal blood, amniotic fluid, and fetal blood. By the 16th day after amalgam placement, accumulations of mercury were found in all analyzed tissues in mothers and babies. In the unborn babies, the highest levels of mercury were in the liver and pituitary gland. The tissue mercury levels continued to increase throughout the course of the investigation. The levels of mercury found in blood and urine were not predictive of the amount found in body tissues.

Although these dental mercury distribution studies were attacked and derided by the dental establishment, they were quickly confirmed by other medical scientists using entirely different research protocols. In Denmark, Danscher and associates placed occlusal amalgam fillings in three vervet monkeys. In three other monkeys, amalgam was implanted in the maxillary bone. Three untreated monkeys served as controls. After one year it was found that the amalgam fillings (total weight 0.7-1.2 grams) caused deposition of mercury in the spinal ganglia, anterior pituitary, adrenal, medulla, liver, kidneys, lungs, and intestinal lymph glands. In monkeys with the maxillary bone implants (total weight 0.1-0.3 grams) mercury was found in the same organs except for liver, lungs, and intestinal lymph glands. The organs of the control animals were devoid of any mercury.(44)

At the University of Calgary Medical School, the research team verified the sheep dental mercury distribution data by doing a similar experiment using a wild-caught monkey. The monkey as a research model is considered to more closely parallel expected human results. Amalgam fillings containing radioactive labelled mercury were placed in the animals teeth. Whole-body tracer images, taken 28 days after placement, revealed similar mercury distribution patterns as those previously reported in sheep. The highest levels of mercury were located in the kidney, gastrointestinal tract, and jaw.(45)

The fetal distribution findings of the Calgary group were also confirmed by a group of Japanese researchers utilizing rats as the study animals. Takahashi and his colleagues found that the mercury concentration in the fetal tissues tended to increase with the increasing number of amalgam fillings in the mother rats.(46)

Additional data regarding fetal effects of dental mercury was presented at the annual meeting of the Society of Toxicology held in Seattle, Washington on 24 February 1992. In one study done at the University of Lund in Sweden, pregnant monkeys exposed to mercury vapor experienced early abortion, premature birth, low birth weight and one perinatal death. Of great significance in this study is that the neonatal exposure levels closely parallel the average intra-oral mercury vapor readings obtained in human amalgam bearers. In another study done at the University of Uppsala in Sweden, pregnant rats exposed to mercury during gestation produced offspring that deviated from normal behavior when compared to the controls.(47)

Another study that was presented at the Society of Toxicology meeting, conducted at the National Institute of Environmental Health Sciences, Research Triangle Park, NC, demonstrated reduced fertility among dental assistants with occupational exposure to mercury. The research compared dental assistants working with amalgam to those not working with amalgam. Work practices and office characteristics known to elevate levels of mercury vapor were used to create a mercury hygiene scale. Women who prepared 30 or more amalgams per week and had three or more poor mercury hygiene factors had a probability of conceiving, in any given menstrual cycle, of only 50% of that for the unexposed women.(48)

It is common medical and scientific knowledge, based on known occupational exposures, that mercury can effect kidney function. What was not known or previously demonstrated was whether mercury from amalgam dental fillings was affecting kidney function. In a classic scientific study (immediately attacked by the ADA and FDA as being flawed), the Calgary group produced some very dynamic information confirming that mercury from dental amalgam seriously damaged the kidneys of animals used in the study. Within 30 days after placement of 12 occlusal amalgam fillings in six adult female sheep, there was a 50% impairment of kidney function and by two months after placement this had risen to 60%.(49) Another interesting aspect of this study was the fact that it demonstrated a significantly decreased excretion of albumin in the urine of the sheep. Corroboration of this effect in humans was found unexpectedly in a Swedish study done by Molin and colleagues: "Our study showed statistically significantly higher urinary albumin levels 12 months after amalgam removal in the experimental group as compared with the pre-removal values. The possibility cannot be excluded that this increased urinary albumin level is a result of the amalgam removal."(50)

There are many research studies in progress around the world that are evaluating the effects of dental mercury on human health. The most recent to be published (April 1993) is a study conducted at three major North American universities that assessed the effect of swallowed or inhaled dental mercury on the normal microflora of the mouth and intestines. The researchers found that within 10 days after placement of mercury-containing fillings in the teeth of the animals, a large percentage of the normal oral and intestinal bacteria had become mercury resistant. When bacteria become mercury resistant they cause the conversion of the different forms of mercury into elemental mercury vapor, which is then recycled back into the body. Of greater

24

immediate concern to the medical profession was the determination that mercury resistant bacteria are also resistant to one or more antibiotics. Antibiotic resistance is a growing problem of great significance to the medical profession in their ability to successfully treat bacterial infections.(51) The results of these bacteriological studies bring into question more of the conclusions concerning dental amalgam safety contained in the Public Health Service Report on Dental Amalgam.(41)

IN SPITE OF ALL OF THE STUDIES OUTLINED SO FAR, THE ADA STILL MAINTAINS THAT THERE IS NO SCIENTIFIC EVIDENCE DEMONSTRATING THAT MERCURY FROM DENTAL AMALGAM CAUSES ANY HEALTH PROBLEMS EXCEPT IN THOSE INDIVIDUALS SENSITIVE TO MERCURY.

While the dental profession continues to ignore the dangers of mercury, the medical profession is becoming more aware and concerned about the harmful effects of mercury on the environment and human health. This was evidenced by the fact that during their December 1992 meeting, the American Medical Association (AMA) House of Delegates passed Resolution 418 submitted by the Michigan Delegation wherein it was: "RESOLVED that the American Medical Association work to establish appropriate federal standards to achieve elimination of lead, mercury and benzene from common household and workplace products." One "workplace" product that the AMA must ultimately concern themselves about is the approximate 50 tons of mercury used annually by dentistry in the production of "silver" amalgam which is then implanted into human teeth.

Scientific research has already demonstrated that mercury, even in small amounts, can damage the brain, heart, lungs, liver, kidneys, thyroid gland, pituitary gland, adrenal glands, blood cells, enzymes and hormones, and suppresses the body's immune (defense) system. In addition, mercury has been shown to pass the placental membrane in pregnant women and cause permanent damage to the brain of a developing baby.

Now let's look at the symptoms of MERCURY TOXICITY contained in medical literature and textbooks (36,52-53):

ELEMENTAL MERCURY VAPOR EXPOSURE

1. PSYCHOLOGICAL DISTURBANCES (Erethism):

Irritability
Nervousness
Shyness or timidity
Loss of memory
Lack of attention
Loss of self-confidence
Decline of intellect
Lack of self control
Fits of anger
Depression
Anxiety
Drowsiness
Insomnia

2. ORAL CAVITY DISORDERS:

Bleeding gums
Alveolar bone loss
Loosening of teeth
Excessive salivation
Foul breath
Metallic taste
Leukoplakia (white patches)
Gingivitis (inflammation of the gums)
Stomatitis (mouth inflammation)
Ulceration of gingiva, palate, tongue
Burning sensation in mouth or throat
Tissue pigmentation

3.GASTROINTESTINAL EFFECTS:

Abdominal cramps

Constipation or diarrhea
Gastrointestinal problems including colitis

4.SYSTEMIC EFFECTS:

CARDIOVASCULAR:
Irregular Heartbeat (tachycardia, bradycardia)
Feeble and irregular pulse
Alterations in blood pressure
Pain or pressure in chest.

NEUROLOGICAL:
Chronic or frequent headaches
Dizziness
Ringing or noises in ears
Fine tremors (hands, feet, lips, eyelids, tongue)

RESPIRATORY:
Persistent cough,
Emphysema
Shallow and irregular respiration

IMMUNOLOGICAL:
Allergies
Asthma
Rhinitis (inflammation of the nose)
Sinusitis
Lymphadenopathy, especially cervical (neck)

ENDOCRINE:
Subnormal temperature
Cold, clammy skin, especially hands and feet
Excessive perspiration

OTHER:
Muscle weakness
Speech disorders
Dim or double vision
Fatigue
Anemia
Hypoxia (lack of oxygen)
Edema (swelling)

Loss of appetite (anorexia)
Loss of weight
Joint pains

5. SEVERE CASES:

Hallucinations
Manic depression

ORGANIC MERCURY EXPOSURE

1. EARLIEST SYMPTOMS:

Fatigue
Headache
Forgetfulness
Inability to concentrate
Apathy
Depression
Outbursts of anger
Decline of intellect

2. LATER FINDINGS:

Numbness and tingling of hands, feet, lips
Muscle weakness progressing to paralysis
Dim or restricted vision
Hearing difficulty
Speech disorders
Loss of memory
Incoordination
Emotional instability
Dermatitis
Renal damage (kidney)
General central nervous system dysfunctions

Most of the symptoms listed above were derived from evaluation of people who had suffered from either chronic or acute industrial exposure or ecological exposure to mercury. The study of micromercurialism, low level exposure, has been very limited in scientific literature. However, there is sufficient evidence to suggest that continual exposure to small doses of mercury over long periods of time, can produce many of the above symptoms. After all, the same biochemical pathways in the human physiology that, when effected by larger doses of mercury result in clinically observable symptoms, are also affected by low continuous mercury exposure regardless of the source. Since inorganic mercury in some body tissues (e.g. brain) has a half life of over 25 years (i.e. it takes the body 25 years to get rid of 1/2 of a single dose) it is only a matter of time and degree of exposure until some form of symptomatology appears.(54)

Unfortunately, mercury is so toxic to the human organism that there can be cell death or irreversible chemical damage long before clinically observable symptoms appear indicating that something is wrong. Further, you could be experiencing some of the symptoms of the mercury released from amalgam dental fillings but since the mercury exposure is so gradual and because the time between the placement of the fillings and the onset of the symptoms can vary so dramatically (from days to years, based on your own biochemical makeup and sensitivity) it may not be readily apparent or identifiable as being associated with dental mercury. Under these conditions your physician would have extreme difficulty in relating subclinical symptoms (not readily apparent or identifiable as being associated with a particular disease or health problem) to mercury toxicity.(55-56) This is not a new hypothesis, Alfred stock the distinguished German chemist said it in 1926 "The dentists are seldom in a position to recognize general effects of amalgam fillings or even learn about them. Patients suffering from nervousness, intellectual exhaustion, catarrh etc. usually do not complain to the dentist. In addition, they are prevented from talking during the treatment. They will rather discuss their problems with the family physician, neurologist, laryngologist and internist."(57)

The same difficulty in diagnosis exists within the dental profession with regard to periodontal disease. Traditionally, simple periodontal disease (periodontitis) has been related to a variety of local irritants, such as subgingival plaque formation, impaction of food, and rough edges of fillings. However, the textbooks and scientific literature establish that mercury and/or amalgam fillings can pathologically damage periodontal tissue. Further, some of the symptoms shown previously under "2. Oral Cavity Disorders" are considered classical symptoms of mercury toxicity.(58-59) Unfortunately, very few periodontists or dentists recognize mercury from dental amalgam fillings as an etiological (causing) factor in the development of periodontal disease.

Will replacing amalgam dental fillings improve an individual's health and reduce overall health care costs? That is a question to which the Health Insurance Bureau in Stockholm, Sweden wanted an answer. To find out, a study was done with 308 patients most of whom had a multiple symptom clinical picture, each with about nine different symptoms. Those patients who exchanged all of their amalgam dental fillings (for non-mercury fillings) reported an improvement of all health symptoms. Generalized symptoms like tiredness, headache and muscle pains improved considerably. Patients in the study had averaged 65 days of sick leave the year prior to amalgam removal. Two years after amalgam exchange this was reduced 30% to a mean of 44 days of sick leave per year. The Health Insurance Bureau concluded that replacement of amalgam fillings would lead to improved health status, fewer days off for sickness, reduced administrative costs for the insurance system and reduced total costs for society.(60)

The above data should be considered representative rather than unrepresentative of the effects of elimination of mercury-containing dental fillings. The vast majority of individuals who have undergone amalgam replacement and the reduction of their mercury body burden have experienced improvements in health that have ranged from minor to startlingly dramatic. For example the statistics listed below were compiled by the Foundation For Toxic Free Dentistry (FTFD) on **1569** patients from 6 different reports:

SELECTED HEALTH SYMPTOM ANALYSIS OF 1569 PATIENTS BEFORE AND AFTER ELIMINATION OF THEIR MERCURY-CONTAINING DENTAL FILLINGS

% of Total	SYMPTOM	Total No.	No. Improved or Cured	% of Cure or Improvement
14%	ALLERGY	221	196	89%
5%	ANXIETY	86	80	93%
5%	BAD TEMPER	81	68	89%
6%	BLOATING	88	70	88%
6%	BLOOD PRESSURE PROBLEMS	99	53	54%
5%	CHEST PAINS	79	69	87%
22%	DEPRESSION	347	315	91%
22%	DIZZINESS	343	301	88%
45%	FATIGUE	705	603	86%
15%	GASTROINTESTINAL PROBLEMS	231	192	83%
8%	GUM PROBLEMS	129	121	94%
34%	HEADACHES	531	460	87%
3%	MIGRAINE HEADACHES	45	39	87%
12%	INSOMNIA	187	146	78%
10%	IRREGULAR HEARTBEAT	159	139	87%
8%	IRRITABILITY	132	119	90%
17%	LACK OF CONCENTRATION	270	216	80%
6%	LACK OF ENERGY	91	88	97%
17%	MEMORY LOSS	265	193	73%
17%	METALLIC TASTE	260	247	95%
7%	MULTIPLE SCLEROSIS	113	86	76%
8%	MUSCLE TREMOR	126	104	83%
10%	NERVOUSNESS	158	131	83%
8%	NUMBNESS ANYWHERE	118	97	82%
20%	SKIN DISTURBANCES	310	251	81%
9%	SORE THROAT	149	128	86%
6%	TACHYCARDIA	97	68	70%
4%	THYROID PROBLEMS	56	44	79%
12%	ULCERS & SORES (ORAL CAVITY)	189	162	86%
7%	URINARY TRACT PROBLEMS	115	87	76%
29%	VISION PROBLEMS	462	289	63%

The above statistics involve a total of 1569 patients in six different studies: 762 patients utilized the FTFD Patient Adverse Reaction Report to individually report changes in their health directly to the FDA and the FTFD; Dr. Mats Hanson, Ph.D. reported on 519 Swedish patients; Henrik Lichtenberg, D.D.S. of Denmark reported on 100 patients; Pierre LaRose, D.D.S. of Canada reported on 80 patients; Robert L. Siblerud O.D., M.S. reported on 86 patients in Colorado as partial fulfillment of a Ph.D. requirement; and Albert V. Zamm, M.D., FACA, FACP reported on 22 of his patients.(61)

One extremely interesting statistic relates to the incidence of allergies. The recent January 1993 Public Health Service Report on Dental Amalgam states: "Only a small proportion of mercury-sensitized individuals respond adversely to the placement of amalgam restorations. The few case reports of adverse allergic reactions to amalgam involve skin reactions, such as rashes and eczematous lesions..."(41) The ADA maintains that the incidence of allergic reaction to amalgam dental fillings is extremely rare, with only 50 case histories being reported in the literature. Statements of this nature totally ignore valid peer reviewed scientific studies demonstrating an allergic reaction to dental amalgam ranging from 16.5% for non-allergic patients to 44% for fourth year dental students.(30-31) More importantly, as the above symptom analysis demonstrates, **the question is not whether the patient is allergic to dental amalgam but rather the direct causal relationship of mercury/amalgam dental fillings to the development of allergies to food, chemicals, and environmental factors.**

In the FTFD analysis, this is supported by the fact that 14% of the individuals reported some type of allergy and that after replacement of their mercury/amalgam dental fillings, 89% reported their condition had improved or was totally eliminated. If you were to extrapolate this data to the approximately 140 million amalgam bearers in the United States (61), there should be 19.6 million people (14%) with amalgam causally related allergies. Of this number 89% or approximately 17.4 million would have their allergies ameliorate or disappear simply by having

32

their mercury dental fillings exchanged for non-mercury ones.

We attempted to look at this from another perspective by first determining the total number of people in the U.S. with allergies. Although there are no hard data available, the NIH estimates the number to be between 40-50 million. Using the lesser number of 40 million people with allergies, it is estimated that 65% (62) or 26 million of them would be amalgam bearers whose allergies may be causally related to their mercury/amalgam dental fillings.

Individuals who have developed a hypersensitivity (allergy) to mercury may be at much greater risk from exposure to micro doses of mercury vapor escaping from amalgam fillings. There are many ways an individual could become sensitized to mercury. For example, mercury was used quite extensively by the medical profession in anti-fungal preparations, diuretics, antiseptics, brain scans (radioactive mercury), etc. Merthiolate and mercurochrome which are very common "first-aid" items in most households and are still used extensively in hospitals, contain mercury. A recent scientific article from Japan indicated that extensive use of mercurochrome was the primary cause of a high degree of sensitivity to mercury in the Japanese population. Mercury is in many of the foods we eat and it is also contained in a great many over the counter drugs and cosmetics; e.g. some mascaras, solutions used with contact lenses, hemorrhoid preparations, etc. Thus, sensitization to mercury could come from a number of sources.(63-65)

HOW CAN I FIND OUT IF THE MERCURY COMING OUT OF MY FILLING IS HURTING ME OR IF I AM HYPERSENSITIVE TO IT?

That is the biggest question we are confronted with today. Again, there is no easy answer. For years, the ADA maintained that urine and blood tests for mercury content were valid means of determining safe exposure and danger. However, after the July 1984 Workshop on the

Biocompatibility of Metals in Dentistry, the ADA finally agreed with the overwhelming scientific evidence (existent since the early 1960's) indicating that blood and urine tests are invalid for determining toxicity or cellular damage that may be occurring in the body. They do however, indicate an exposure to mercury.

Appendix A details a number of tests that may be helpful in establishing a diagnosis of possible mercury damage.

One of the standard methods utilized by the medical profession to determine hypersensitivity is the use of skin testing. Dilute concentrations of the suspected allergen are applied to the skin by use of a patch (like a band aid) or injected just below the surface of the skin. There is considerable controversy concerning the use of this procedure. One potential problem encountered is that the patch test itself could greatly exacerbate your symptoms and reaction if you are already sensitive to mercury. Another problem stems from the difference of opinion amongst medical allergists and dermatologists as to what type of mercury to test with and how dilute to make the solution. The biggest controversy seems to hinge around what kind of reaction constitutes a positive reaction (allergic). Some say you are positive if the skin turns red and whealed (burning, itching, swelling). Others say there are systemic manifestations such as changes in blood pressure, temperature and pulse.

Regardless of what the correct interpretation of mercury patch testing may be, there are certain individuals who should not allow themselves to be mercury patch tested: Pregnant women, diagnosed cases of Systemic Lupus Erythematosus, Multiple Sclerosis, Amyotrophic Lateral Sclerosis (ALS), Alzheimer's disease, Leukemia, Hodgkins disease, cardiovascular disease, mental illness (especially manic depression), Acrodynia, and MLNS (Kawasaki's disease). Above all, if you suspect you are sensitive to mercury, do not be tested unless considered absolutely necessary.

Perhaps some day a testing protocol will be developed that will satisfy everyone. Until that time though, we believe the questionable results do not warrant the additional exposure.

There are electrical measuring devices, similar to a volt meter or ammeter, that can demonstrate that you have electrical currents in your mouth, but that's all they can do. They have no diagnostic value for determining whether you are at risk or not, although as stated previously these electrical currents are capable of causing unexplained pain, ulcerations, inflammations, etc.

There is another category of electrical device that is diagnostic and operates within the science of acupuncture and energy flow of the meridians. Unfortunately, the FDA has not seen fit to approve this category of instrumentation for use in the United States. Consequently, it is being used primarily to conduct and document research aspects of the discipline. The instruments costs thousands of dollars and require extensive training and study to be used properly. In the hands of a trained clinician it can provide exceptional diagnostic information.(66)

Many scientists and researchers are attempting to find some enzyme system in the body that will permit laboratory evaluation of blood, urine or saliva to show conclusively that mercury is inhibiting that particular enzyme's metabolic function in the body. Although these experiments are exciting, none have proven clinically useful as yet. Recently however, "The Porphyrin Profile Test for Mercury" has been approved. See Appendix A for details.

One instrument which is available is the Jerome mercury vapor analyzer. This instrument can be used to measure the amount of mercury vapor present in the mouth before and after chewing. A reading is taken before the patient is asked to chew sugarless gum for ten minutes, after which another intra-oral reading is taken. Equations have been developed that make it possible to estimate your potential body burden of mercury directly attributable to your mercury-containing dental fillings.(67-69)

The results of mercury vapor readings are excellent for the following reasons:

1. It graphically demonstrates that mercury vapor is coming out of the amalgam fillings and being inhaled.

2. It is known that mercury vapor is a serious poison.

We also know that mercury vapor inhaled into the lungs, is absorbed almost 100 percent, and immediately passes into the bloodstream. In its elemental mercury vapor state it takes approximately four (4) minutes before it is converted or oxidized into an ionic state. While in its elemental form, mercury vapor is lipid (fat) soluble and readily passes through the blood brain barrier or the placental membrane. It can also accumulate in other organs and tissues of the body.(70)

Recent autopsy studies of humans suffering accidental death were done in Germany, Sweden, and the United States. All of these studies showed a positive correlation between the number of amalgam surfaces and fillings in the mouth and the degree of accumulation of mercury in the brain.(33-35)

Complete Blood Count: This is usually a routine blood test prescribed by many physicians. White blood cell count variations (either elevations or depressions) have been found in cases of known mercury poisoning. A study by Eggleston presented preliminary results indicating a possible suppression of the immune system T-lymphocytes by both dental amalgam and dental nickel alloys.(71) More recent studies done at the University of Pennsylvania have clearly demonstrated that mercury-containing compounds adversely effect the immune system; moreover, the decrease in lymphocyte function following exposure to mercury indicates that mercury is immunotoxic at very low exposure levels.(72,73) These lymphocyte and monocyte cells control your body's immunity. Accordingly, such

36

tests could also prove very helpful in arriving at a diagnosis.

Perhaps the single most important diagnostic tool available at the present time is you, the patient. It is extremely important for your dentist to have your complete medical history. You can greatly assist your dentist by making sure that you provide him, or her, with all the details of your medical history. A sample of a specially designed medical history form is enclosed in this booklet. It was designed to help stimulate your memory regarding any medical problems or symptoms you may have had. When you fill out your medical history form, don't hurry. It is extremely important to you and your dentist that you be very thorough. Above all be sure to state whether you have any allergies and whether you specifically have any known allergies to metals or petrochemicals (plastics).

Anyone contemplating having their mercury-containing fillings replaced with non-mercury containing materials should read Appendix A prior to initiating any dental work.

DENTAL MATERIAL OPTIONS WHEN YOU REPLACE AMALGAM.

There are several options available.

Gold has been used in dentistry longer than amalgam and has been shown to be relatively biocompatible. The gold normally used in dentistry is an alloy. This means that it has been mixed with some other metal or element to give it certain structural characteristics. These are usually palladium, copper or cobalt. The actual percentage of gold contained in these alloys will vary from 2 percent to 92 percent depending on the manufacturer and the price range desired. The only problem with gold is that it is expensive and the price normally will fluctuate with the price of gold on the world market. Since it is a metal alloy, the gold used in dentistry still has the capability of participating in the oral galvanism phenomenon. Moreover, cheaper gold alloys often have base metals added. These additional metals could pose problems. A good dentist however, only uses good materials.

The newer materials available on the market today are referred to as bonded resin ceramics, composite resins or just composites. The term "newer materials" refers to those being used to fill or restore the posterior (back) teeth; composite materials have been used for more than 25 years in fillings placed in the anterior (front) teeth that are not subjected to great chewing forces.

The newer posterior composite materials have a much different structural formulation. Although there are several types available, their composition is essentially one of a quartz-filled Bis-GMA resin. From your standpoint as the potential recipient of these materials, unless you happen to be a physicist or engineer, your main concern isn't the actual chemical structure. The more important question is are they safe to put in your mouth or are they going to be as potentially harmful as amalgam?

These new composites being used for posterior restorations have been subjected to hundreds of research experiments all over the world to determine whether they were biocompatible and safe to use in the human body. To date, the data produced by these studies indicates a very high degree of biocompatibility, when properly placed.(74,75) A key feature of composite plastics is their extremely large molecular size, which prevents penetration of body cells. However, some composites contain elements such as aluminum, that are potentially harmful if they are not bound into the material.

There has been one problem however with the use of the new composites and that is post operative pain and sensitivity. There is a small percentage of people receiving composite restorations that experience varying degrees of post operative pain and thermal sensitivity (hot or cold). Although millions of composite restorations have been placed, the profession is very concerned about those individuals who experience this post operative condition.

Research into this phenomenon is clearly showing that the use of these new materials is very technique sensitive. This means the dentist must be well informed on the different materials - i.e. bases, cements, composites - and their proper use. Some of the earlier materials that were being placed in direct contact with the dentin, to seal it, appear to have been irritating to the pulp and may have been causing varying degrees of post operative pain and sensitivity problems in some individuals. However, research and patient experience is now showing that the use of glass ionomer cements and certain calcium hydroxide products being placed as a base over the exposed dentin have been very successful in eliminating or reducing this problem.

Some people however may still experience an initial sensitivity to hot or cold that will dissipate over time. During this period your dentist may recommend the use of certain desensitizing tooth pastes. However, if the pain or sensitivity persists you should advise your dentist. This is true for any dental procedure regardless of the type of material that was placed in your mouth; i.e., gold, composite, etc. We are all biochemically individual, which means that you could possibly react to something that normally doesn't cause any problems in other people. Remember, your dentist can't help you if he doesn't know a problem exists.

No material is perfect for everyone. The potential for reaction exists for any foreign material implanted into the body. To further delineate what dental materials you may be sensitive to, some dentists advocate using sensitivity or biocompatability testing. This type of testing is intended to demonstrate the various materials that are best suited for you. Although these tests are still controversial in the dental and medical professions, they may be worthy of consideration for patients with severe illnesses or compromised immune systems.(76) Additional information can be obtained by calling (719) 550-0008. Another option that some dentists are using is the placement of temporary or interim fillings. In these situations, whether for personal health or financial reasons, mercury-containing fillings are temporarily (6-12 months) replaced with glass ionomer fillings. These are then replaced with more permanent materials as health or finances permit.

How long will composite materials last? The newer composites being used haven't been around long enough to have been subjected to 10, 15, or 20 year longitudinal studies. However, there are several 5-7 year studies that indicate wear characteristics that are as good if not better than amalgam. Although the final jury might still be out, all present indications are good. In this regard, there are several aspects of these new materials that are very encouraging:

(1) They do not contain mercury.

(2) They are esthetically pleasing. When you smile, people do not see black, grey, or silver areas. All they see is what looks like natural tooth color. In fact, you're hard pressed to tell the difference between the composite and your own natural teeth.

(3) They do not generate any electrical currents and therefore do not participate in helping to corrode any other metallic fillings or restorations you may have in your mouth.

(4) There is less loss of your natural tooth structure because the dentist doesn't have to do extensive preparation for the new materials.

(5) The end product using these materials can truly be called restorations rather than fillings. Amalgam doesn't restore anything. Composites are bonded to remaining tooth structure, are thermally insulating and with the bases and bonding agents used to place the composite, there is much more protection for the pulp and enamel structure of the tooth. In fact, there is scientific evidence indicating that tooth strength increases and that the tooth can be restored to up to 98 percent of its original predecayed state.

Today, there is a much wider selection of materials available in dentistry that can be used as suitable alternatives to the use of metal. For example there are products available that are heat and pressure cured, which imparts different structural and finishing properties to the final product. Normally this is done in a dental laboratory. These types of materials are excellent for metal free crowns and for cosmetic dentistry applications such as very thin laminates that can be bonded to your teeth (with little or, in some cases, no tooth preparation) to cover bad stains, or to cover diastemas (spaces between teeth). There are also porcelain laminates and veneers being used for cosmetic applications; and there are also metal free ceramic and/or glass crowns available.

The trend in dentistry moves more and more towards being totally metal free. There is now a metal-free partial denture material available. These flouropolymer thermoplastic materials are chemically inert and possess remarkable stability. If you are a partial denture appliance wearer you may wish to discuss this new type of partial with your dentist.

Unfortunately, and for far too long, dentistry has had to rely on and utilize potentially toxic metals in the oral environment because there were not any acceptable alternatives available. Now, however, the new technology and scientific advances that have been made are providing a variety of non-metal materials that can be used instead of the traditional metals. So you see, there are a multitude of options available for you to consider.

IS REPLACING AMALGAMS DANGEROUS?

That depends on who you ask. If you ask the ADA they will say yes. Their official position published in the January 1984 issue of the ADA news and again in the JADA in September of 1984 is "The Association wishes to emphasize that, except in individuals sensitive to mercury, there is no reason why a patient should seek at this time to have amalgam restorations (silver fillings)

41

removed. Indeed, the effect of such a procedure and further restorative operations could be detrimental to the patient's oral health, including the unnecessary loss of teeth, and cannot be justified."(2,26) The ADA official position in 1992 is still the same.

The second sentence may very well be true - if the dentist removing the amalgam is not aware of the dangers of mercury exposure and well trained and qualified in the procedures to protect the patient. The facts of the matter are:

(1) Dentists routinely remove amalgam fillings every day and replace them with other amalgam fillings. So I assume what the ADA is saying is that it is all right to replace amalgam with amalgam, but it is harmful to replace amalgam with composite.

(2) The average life of an amalgam filling is 5.5 to 11.5 years.(77) In six year old children the average survival time for occlusal amalgam fillings was twenty-six months.(78) Most fillings are replaced because of decay under the filling, excessive corrosion, fracture, etc. The procedure is so commonplace, that the insurance companies will pay for replacement of an amalgam filling after only one year.

(3) The primary risks to a patient's health are the competence of the dentist and statements being made by the ADA that cannot be supported with primary scientific research. There are certainly situations beyond the control of your dentist which may cause you to lose a tooth. However, the newer materials are so much more flexible and advantageous to work with that in many instances, teeth can be saved that would otherwise be lost if amalgam was the only material available.

There are special techniques utilized by your dentist to remove amalgam fillings. If done properly, there is minimum exposure to increased levels of mercury vapor caused by the removal procedure. However, we feel it important that you, the patient, should be aware of certain aspects related to amalgam removal:

(1) The dentist should have an assistant present to assist in minimizing their exposure, and yours, to any mercury vapor. The correct protocol requires the use of high volumes of cold water both from the drill and separate irrigation by the assistant, who should also be simultaneously using high volume suction evacuation of the vapor and particles resulting from the removal procedure. The assistant should hold the high volume evacuator positioned next to the tooth being worked on until all of the cut filling and cavity have been cleaned out. A new aspirating device, invented in Sweden, and soon to be marketed in the U.S. goes a long way to solve many of the common amalgam filling removal and replacement problems. This device called Clean-Up^{TM} is a high volume plastic evacuator that fits directly over the tooth being worked on. This provides continuous evacuation of the work area during the entire removal procedure. It can also be used during the composite placement process to keep areas dry when it is critical to proper placement.(79) Available from Future Dentistry, Inc. (800)-282-9670.

(2) It is the volatility of mercury that necessitates all the precautions and correct techniques. Mercury vapor pressure doubles with every ten degree centigrade rise in temperature. One acceptable procedure that minimizes extensive grinding (which generates great temperature increases) involves sectioning the amalgam into chunks versus just grinding it out.

(3) In some dental offices the dentist may ask you to breathe through a nose piece that will permit you to draw air from another area of the operatory.

(4) During amalgam removal, the dentist and assistant are at greater risk from exposure to mercury aerosol spray and vapor. They will be wearing special clothing, masks and surgical gloves. These actions protect them from excessive exposure to mercury during repeated removal operations.

(5) Some dentists will utilize a rubber dam during the amalgam removal procedure. This is a square of latex rubber stretched on a frame. It isolate the tooth or teeth being worked on. The rubber dam is supposed to prevent the patient from swallowing ground out amalgam particles and accidentally inhaling mercury fumes. However, high levels of mercury vapor have been measured under the rubber dam, therefore if your dentist does use the rubber dam, you should not breathe through your mouth during the removal process.

(6) The office and operatory should be well ventilated. In this regard, many mercury-free dentists are now installing central vacuuming systems in their offices. You may be asked to hold the vacuum hose on your chest during the removal process. This provides an additional high vacuum suction source, drawing out mercury vapor and mercury aerosol generated during the removal process. Mercury vapor analyzer testing of this additional safeguard has shown it to dramatically reduce mercury contamination outside the body.

(7) Don't be in a hurry. Current information indicates that it is better to replace only a few amalgams at a time, with several weeks in between appointments. Regardless of the precautions outlined, some individuals may experience reactions to the mercury released during the removal procedures. These are described as being flu-like and can last from one to seven days. Symptoms may include fever, nausea, headaches, etc. If these symptoms persist, please let your dentist know.

"Sequential removal" of amalgam fillings is a controversial technique advocated by some dentists. Sequential removal requires the dentist to measure and chart the electrical current of each filling and to remove/and or replace the amalgam fillings based on the charted information starting with the highest negative readings first. There is no scientific data to support the use of sequential removal. More importantly, there is absolutely no scientific data to support the statements being made by the proponents of sequential removal that "if your dentist doesn't use sequential removal it will cause the mercury to remain locked into the tissues." Moreover, it has been well established scientifically that precise measurement of these electrical potentials is not possible. Measurements are of specific points on the fillings, not the entire fillings which, therefore, cannot be compared to each other.

However, if your dentist has the equipment and wants to replace your amalgam fillings sequentially, there is no problem in allowing him or her to do so. Just bear in mind that it is not a prerequisite for successful amalgam replacement. In fact, most dentists around the world replace fillings by quadrant, usually starting with the quadrant that has the largest fillings, thus removing the largest source of mercury first.

There are other steps your dentist will probably recommend to minimize or reduce the potential for aggravating any existing mercury related symptomatology or, for that matter, causing any problems if you are symptom free. These are normally nutritional and involve diet modification and taking certain supplements. The reasons are to reduce your exposure to mercury sources other than amalgam dental fillings and to assist your body in coping with any exposure directly related to the removal procedure. (For complete information on this subject read the Bio-Probe book entitled "Dental Mercury Detox")

Diet modification usually involves attempting to reduce the amount of mercury ingested from dietary sources by elimination or reduction of certain types of fish and other foods that normally have a high mercury content. Reduction of refined carbohydrates and sugars is also beneficial, as oral and gut bacteria seem to thrive on these types of food. Increasing dietary fiber intake is also helpful by inducing a faster transit time of waste matter and toxins to be excreted, as is increasing or insuring that there is an adequate water intake to assist the body in flushing toxins through the kidneys.

The nutritional supplements your dentist may recommend are those that scientific research has shown to either bind with the mercury and help your body excrete it or help your body to neutralize some of the biochemical byproducts created when mercury affects normal metabolic processes. This is a very dynamic area of research producing new data continuously. We won't list the nutrients and function, but leave that aspect of overall amalgam removal protocol to your dentist or physician (should you be under the care of one who has prescribed amalgam removal because of suspected mercury toxicity).

There are also therapeutic chelating protocols available. DMSA and DMPS are well established mercury chelating agents that have used in European countries for many years. They should be used only by qualified physicians. An additional benefit is that they may be utilized diagnostically (urine mercury mobilization or challenge test) to firmly establish a body burden of mercury.

The medical text book "Environmental and Occupational Medicine"(80) indicates that sweat induction may also be of therapeutic value in reducing the total body burden of mercury. The Spanish use sweat therapy on workers in the mercury mines who exhibit signs or symptoms of mercury vapor toxicity. Any means of inducing sweating would appear to be acceptable; i.e., steam baths, saunas, heat lamps, exercise, etc. Using this type of sweat therapy increases the elimination of mercury through the skin and should therefore help in reducing the total body burden. NOTE: Pregnant women or anyone with a history of cardiovascular problems should obtain approval from their physician prior to undertaking routine sweat therapy.

HOW EXPENSIVE ARE THE NEW MATERIALS AND WILL MY INSURANCE PLAN PAY FOR THEM?

At the present time the price that the dentist must pay for these new materials is more than he would have paid for the amalgam. Coupled to this higher material cost is a very technique sensitive procedure to place the restoration that, as a general rule, will require the dentist to spend more time with you to properly place and bond the material to your tooth. A recent research study of this particular factor showed that composite resin restorations required 35 percent more placement time than did the amalgam fillings.(81) The net result is a higher unit cost per surface for composite restorations versus amalgam fillings.

Fine, most people would have no problem in understanding the equation: higher costs of non-metal restoration raw materials and more time expended to complete the restoration procedures equals a higher unit cost than amalgam. Reasonable and fair assumption? WRONG. At least in the case of the insurance companies it appears to be wrong, because certain insurance companies are not allowing fair value reimbursement for the placement of composites.

The end result of this lack of understanding is total confusion, as some insurance companies will pay only the comparable cost for an amalgam filling. This means that the patient has to pay the difference in cost between amalgam and composite.

The basis for non-payment has previously been that the ADA had not approved any composites for use in posterior teeth. That situation is changing, but in ways that are difficult to understand. According to an article in "The Dental Advisor" Vol. 8, No. 4, December 1991, the ADA has given Restricted Use (wear not to exceed 125 micrograms after two years and 175 micrograms after four years) approval to at least ten different posterior composites. However, composites having previously received provisional or full acceptance by the ADA are now approved only for restricted use. Even stranger, no composite has been approved for "Unrestricted Use" although several of them have wear rates that approach that of amalgam and are much less than the 25 micrograms per year established by the ADA to qualify for approval and placement in the "Unrestricted Use" category.

It would appear that the ADA has an agenda for non-approval that embraces reasons other than product quality and acceptability. It is probably not just a coincidence that the dental establishments in several countries maintain that they will immediately replace the use of amalgam when suitable posterior composites are available. We think it important that you realize that the American Dental Association is a trade organization in which membership is strictly voluntary and, by its own admission, has no regulatory authority over what materials a dentist may use or not use.(82)

There is also a much more serious situation that exists. This involves the patient whose own physician (medical doctor) has determined that the individual was sensitive to mercury or possibly suffering from mercury toxicity and has written a prescription to have all the amalgams replaced with gold or composite. Some insurance companies are refusing to pay for complete replacement of amalgam fillings even when the patient presents documentation from medical doctors stating categorically that the patient's health requires such action to be taken. These companies are refusing to pay under medical or dental coverage, citing as the basis for their refusal that there is no scientific data to support taking such action. Presumably, the insurance carriers are relying on recently issued policy statements of the ADA that, although research is demonstrating the release of mercury vapor from amalgam fillings, the quantities released do not pose a health threat. There is no scientific data to support the position taken by the ADA. Conversely, even recent medical text books are now recognizing micromercurialsm as a disease syndrome whose three primary symptoms are: increased excitability, tremors, and gingivitis.(83)

In summary there are several things wrong with the positions being taken by the insurance companies and the ADA:

1. The ADA is a trade organization and has no legal or regulatory authority to dictate what products a dentist may or may not use.

2. The insurance companies have no legal authority to discourage the use of composites for restorative dental work and insist that they will only pay for the placement of a known poison in your mouth. In fact, based on current scientific data, by doing so they may well be dramatically increasing their own liability. 3. The ADA, the insurance company or, for that matter, the dentist do not have the right to deny an "informed" individual his/her right to freedom of choice.

4. It is ultimately the decision of the dentist as to what material will best accomplish the operative procedures that must be done, (providing you have signed an informed consent agreement). This principle was recently reaffirmed by the Swedish Supreme Court.(84) Insurance companies have no legal right to determine the diagnosis and treatment of patients.

5. More and more research data is being published demonstrating the intra-oral release of mercury vapor from mercury-containing dental fillings under a variety of actual conditions that are normally encountered. It appears from the data that each individual condition - i.e., chewing, drinking hot fluids, bruxing, tooth brushing, etc. - is capable of stimulating a sufficient release of mercury vapor that temporarily exceeds existing control standards. Moreover, current research taking into consideration the continual static unstimulated release of mercury vapor from silver/mercury dental fillings together with the stimulated release, establishes this as the predominant contribution to human exposure to mercury vapor.(12,40) That being the case, it is irresponsible for any organization or individual to make any claim that the amount of mercury vapor being released intra-orally and inhaled is insufficient to pose a threat to health. This is especially so when a physician has determined that the patient may be at risk and has requested that the silver/mercury fillings be replaced.

6. Serious consideration must be given by all concerned to the potential that mercury escaping from silver/mercury dental fillings may, in some instances, be a primary etiological factor (cause) involved in initiation of the periodontal disease. Most medical diagnostic, toxicological, and historical descriptions of mercury toxicity list stomatitis (inflammation of the mouth) or gingivitis (inflammation of the gums) as one of the three most prevalent signs or symptoms of mercury poisoning.

Consequently, there are two aspects of this problem that must be addressed in regard to insurance payment for silver/mercury filling replacement: 1) If the patient has periodontal involvement and amalgam fillings, the dentist (and physician if solely under medical care) must be able to scientifically prove that mercury escaping from the amalgam fillings is not the cause of the periodontal problem. Failure to consider this possible etiological factor (especially in the light of the historical identification of mercury as a cause of this disease in cases of toxicity) presents both moral and legal issues of great import; and 2) Documentation of the periodontal condition, along with the identification of mercury as the "probable cause", should be sufficient grounds for insurance prepayment approval of proposed dental treatment plans requiring the replacement of amalgams as one of the desired therapeutics of choice to treat the disease condition. Refusal by the insurance carrier to approve such recommended procedures could be legally indefensible.

7. Individuals with kidney problems should be considered as candidates for elimination of chronic mercury exposure.

8. As a final note, we have not differentiated between children and adults in our discussions. However, authoritative texts state that children are more vulnerable to the potential harmful effects of mercury vapor than adults because of the dose/body weight relationships. The dose a 150 pound adult might accommodate, could be devastating to a 75 pound child. Consequently, under no condition that we can envisage, should children be

subjected to the placement of amalgams. Insurance carriers do not take this into consideration.

Appendix A outlines a variety of tests that are available that may serve as a basis to refute intractable positions taken by your insurance carrier or, all else failing, provide the basis for other appropriate action.

CHECK THE COVERAGE PROVIDED BY YOUR INSURANCE POLICY

If your insurance company will not pay full price for composite restorations then register a written complaint with your State Insurance Commissioner, your employer, your union representative (if appropriate) and the insurance company. Urge your employer to shop around for another carrier who will provide full coverage for biocompatible non-metal restorative materials and procedures and who does not arbitrarily or capriciously seek to deny or eliminate your constitutional right to freedom of choice.

Should you be refused payment on a presubmittal claim related to amalgam replacement for health reasons, you may wish to consider having your attorney write a letter to your insurance carrier requesting that they have their corporate attorney respond in writing indicating the claim denial and stating that the insurance carrier assumes all liability for health problems that may result from the continued release of mercury vapor from the silver/mercury dental material that you presently have in your mouth.

WHAT IS INFORMED CONSENT?

Included as an appendix to this booklet is a sample of a form entitled Informed Consent. It has been designed to be utilized in conjunction with this booklet. One of the primary purposes of this booklet is to reduce the tremendous amount of time the doctor must spend in providing information to the patient concerning the very complex relationship between mercury amalgam fillings, the release of mercury vapor from amalgam fillings, some of the physiological considerations associated with the phenomenon and the position of the American Dental Association on the overall safety of mercury amalgam as a dental material.

The intent of all this effort is to insure that you, the patient, have sufficient information upon which to make an independent judgement as to whether you; 1) wish to have any more mercury amalgam placed in your teeth, 2) should actively consider having all of your mercury amalgam fillings replaced with the new composite materials or gold, and 3) are comfortable with the fact that the composite materials being used are adequate and that research has shown them to be biocompatible when placed properly.

Perhaps the most important aspect of informed consent relates to the fact that at this point in time, based on the scientific research that has been done, you as a patient understand that no claims can be made that removal and replacement of mercury amalgam fillings will cure any known disease or eliminate or modify any signs or symptoms of any disease or disease syndrome that you may have. Although there are hundreds of scientific reports dealing with the toxicity of mercury to humans there has not been any "scientifically reliable" published research studies that clearly ties elemental mercury vapor from dental amalgams to a specific disease or disease syndrome. There are however, a tremendous number of case histories (clinical evidence) that attest to the therapeutic efficacy of mercury amalgam replacement. Although we are routinely subjected to mercury intake from the environment and our food chain, these are sources essentially beyond our control. However, replacement of amalgams is within our individual control and does reduce our total daily mercury intake by an amount usually equal to or greater than that received from dietary or environmental sources. The informed consent agreement is a two-way street, it insures that you are informed and at the same time insures that the dentist has informed you of all aspects of the proposed dental treatment plan and has answered whatever questions you may have had.

REFERENCES

1. Bremmer, D.K. The Story of Dentistry (3rd ed.), 1954. Dental Items of Interest Publishing Co., Inc., Brooklyn, NY.
2. ADA News. Editorial and accompanying patient handout on the safety of dental amalgam. Jan. 2, 1984.
3. ADA Pamphlet Number W186. Dental amalgam filling dental health care needs. 1985.
4. When your patients ask about dental amalgam. JADA 122, August 1991.
5. Pleva J. Mercury from dental amalgams; exposure and effects. Int J Risk & Safety in Med. 3:1-22, 1992.
6. Council on Dental Materials, Instruments, and Equipment. Recommendations in dental mercury hygiene, 1984. JADA. 109:617-619, October 1984.
7. Svare, C.W. Dental Amalgam Related Mercury Vapor Exposure. Cal Dent Assoc J. pp 55-60, Oct. 1984.
8. Vimy, M.J. and Lorscheider, F.L. Intra-Oral Air Mercury Released From Dental Amalgam. J. Dent Res. Vol 64:1069-1071, August 1985.
9. Vimy M.J. and Lorscheider, F.L. Intra-Oral Air Mercury: Estimation of Daily Dose From Dental Amalgam. J. Dent. Res. Vol 65:1072-1075, August 1985.
10. Emler B.F. and Cardone M. Sr. An Assessment of Mercury in Mouth Air. J. Dent. Res. Vol 64:247, IADR Abstract No. 652, 1985.
11. Patterson J.E., Weissberg B.G. and Dennison P.J. Mercury In Human Breath From Dental Amalgams. Bull. Environ Contam Toxicol. 34:459-468, 1985.
12. IPCS (International Programme On Chemical Safety) Environmental Health Criteria 118 Inorganic Mercury. Page 36, 1991. Published under the joint sponsorship of the United Nations Environment Programme, the International Labour Organisation, and the World Health Organization.
13. Aposhian HV; Bruce DC; Alter W; Dart RC; Hurlbut KM; and Aposhian MM. Urinary mercury after administration of 2,3-dimercaptopropane-1-sulfonic acid: correlation with dental amalgam score. FASEB J. 6:2472-2476, 1992.
14. Zander D; Ewers U; Freier I; Brockhaus. Studies on human exposure to mercury. 3. DMPS induced mobilization of mercury in subjects with and without amalgam fillings. Zentralblatt fur Hygiene und Umwelmedizin 192(5):447-454, Feb 1992.
15. Skare I. (Swedish National Board of Occupational Safety and Health). Mercury exposure from amalgam - a background study. Abstr Scand Occup Hyg Mtg. Iceland. Aug 1987.
16. Skare I and Engvist A. Amalgam restorations - an important source to human exposure of mercury and silver. LÄKARTIDNINGEN 15:1299-1301, 1992.
17. WHO task group on evaluation of certain food additives and contaminants. Geneva: World Health Organization, 1972. (WHO Technical Report Series No 505).
18. Stock A and Cucuel F. Der Quecksilbergehalt der menschlichen Ausscheidungen und des menschlichen Blutes. Z Angew Chemie 47:641-647, 1934.
19. Frykholm KO. Mercury from dental amalgam. Uppsala: Almqvist & Wiskell, 1957.
20. Störtebecker P. Mercury Poisoning from Dental Amalgam -a Hazard to Human Brain. Page 32-43, 1985. Bio-Probe, Inc. P.O. Box 608010, Orlando, FL 32860-8010.
21. Summers AO., et al. Mercury released from dental "silver" fillings increases the incidence of multiply resistant bacteria in the oral and intestinal normal flora. 1991 Annual meeting, American Society For Microbiology. Dallas, TX May 5-9, 1991. Abstract A137.

22. Schriever W. and Diamond L.E. Electromotive forces and electric currents caused by metallic dental fillings. J Dent Res. Vol 31(2):205-228, 1952.

23. Schneider PE, Sarker NK. Mercury release from dispersalloy amalgam. IADR Abstract #630, 1982.

24. Hyams B.L. and Ballon H.C. Dissimilar metals in the mouth as a possible cause of otherwise unexplainable symptoms. Can Med Assoc J. Vol XXIXX:488-491, 1933.

25. Phillips R.W. Skinner's Science of Dental Materials. (7th ed) W.B. Saunders Co. Philadelphia, 1973.

26. NIDR Workshop: Biocompatibility of metals in dentistry. JADA Vol 109(3):469-471, 1984.

27. Viola PL and Cassano GB. The effect of chlorine on mercury vapor intoxication. Autoradiographic study. Med. Lavoro 59:437-444, 1968.

28. Cremer F. (Ed.), Die Fabrikation der Silber- und Quecksilber-Spiegel. Hartlebens Verl., Wien u. Leipzig 1904.

29. Viola PL. L'influenza del cloro sull'intossicazione da vapori di mercurio. Med. Lavoro 58:60-65, 1967.

30. Djerassi E. and Berova N. The possibilities of allergic reactions from silver amalgam restorations. Int Dent J. 19(4):481-488, 1969.

31. Miller E.G., Perry W.L. and Wagner M.J. Prevalence of mercury hypersensitivity in dental students. J Prosthetic Dent. 58(2):235-237, Aug 1987.

32. ADA. When your patients ask about mercury in amalgam. JADA. 120:395-8. April 1990.

33. Schiele R. et al. Studies on the mercury content in brain and kidney related to number and condition of amalgam fillings. Inst Occup & Social Med. Univ Erlangen-Nurnberg. Symposium March 12, 1984, Cologne. Amalgam-Viewpoints from Medicine and Dental Medicine.

34. Friberg L. et al. Mercury in the central nervous system in relation to amalgam fillings. LÄKARTIDNINGEN 83(7):519-522, 1986.

35. Eggleston D.W. and Nylander M. Correlation of dental amalgam with mercury in brain tissue. J Prosthetic Dent. 58(6):704-707, Dec 1987.

36. Hanson M. Mercury Bibliography (3rd Edition) 285 symptoms of mercury toxicity and 12000 mercury citations. Bio-Probe, Inc. P.O. Box 608010, Orlando, FL 32860-8010.

37. Wenstrup D; Ehmann WD; and Markesbery WR. Trace element imbalances in isolated subcellular fractions of Alzheimer's disease brains. Brain Research, 533:125-131, 1990.

38. Duhr E; Pendergrass C; Kasarkis J; Slevin J; and Haley B. Hg^{2+} induces GTP-Tubulin interactions in rat brain similar to those observed in Alzheimer's disease. FASEB, 75th Annual Meeting, April 21-25, 1991 Atlanta, Georgia, Abstract 493.

39. The Alzheimer's Disease Research Center Update Newsletter, Fall 1991, University of Kentucky, Lexington, Kentucky.

40. Clarkson T.W., Friberg L., Hursh J.B. and Nylander M. The prediction of intake of mercury vapor from amalgams. In: Biological Monitoring of Toxic Metals. Plenum Press, NY, 1988.

41. DENTAL AMALGAM: A scientific review and recommended Public Health Service strategy for research, education and regulation. January 1993, Department of Health and Human Services, Public Health Service.

42. Hahn, LJ; Kloiber; R; Vimy; MJ; Takahashi, Y: Lorscheider, FL. Dental "silver" fillings: a source of mercury exposure revealed by whole-body image scan and tissue analysis. FASEB J. 3:2641-6. Dec 1989.

43. Vimy, MJ; Takahashi, Y; Lorscheider, Fl. Maternal-fetal distribution of mercury (^{203}Hg) released from dental amalgam fillings. Amer J Physiol. 258:R939-45. April 1990.

44. Danscher G; Hørsted-Bindley P; and Rungby J. Traces of mercury in organs from primates with amalgam fillings. Exp Molecular Path 52:291-299, 1990.

45. Hahn LJ; Kloiber R; Leininger RW; Vimy MJ; and Lorscheider FL. Whole-body imaging of the distribution of mercury released from dental fillings into monkey tissues. FASEB J 4:3256-3260, 1990.

46. Takahashi, Y; Tsuruta S; Hasegawa J; and Kameyama Y. Number of amalgam fillings in pregnant rats and mercury concentration in their fetuses. J Dent Res 71 (IADR Abstracts), page 571, A445, 1992.

47. Berlin M; Hua J; Logdberg B; and Warvinge K. Prenatal exposure to mercury vapor: Effects on brain development. The Toxicologist, 12(1), Abstract 245, 1992.

48. Rowland A; Baird D; Weinber C; Shore D; Shy C; and Wilcox A. The Toxicologist, 12(1), Abstract 246, 1992.

49. Boyd ND; Benediktsson H; Vimy MJ; Hooper DE; and Lorscheider FL. Mercury from dental "silver" tooth fillings impairs sheep kidney function. Am J Physiol 261 (Regulatory Integrative Comp. Physiol. 30): R1010-R1014, 1991.

50. Molin M. et al. Mercury selenium, and glutathione peroxidase before and after amalgam removal in man. Acta Odontol Scand. 48:189-202, 1990.

51. Summers AO; Wireman J; Vimy MJ; Lorscheider FL; Marshall B; Levy SB; Bennett S; Billard L. Mercury released from dental "silver" fillings provokes an increase in mercury and antibiotic resistant bacteria in the primate oral and intestinal flora. Antimicrobial Agents & Chemotherapy, 37:825-834, 1993.

52. Oettingen W.F. Poisoning A Guide to Clinical Diagnosis and Treatment. W.B. Saunders Co., Philadelphia 1958.

53. Environmental Health Criteria 1, Mercury. World Health Organization, Geneva, 1976.

54. Sugita M. The biological half-time of heavy metals. The existence of a third slowest component. Int Arch Occup Health, Vol 41:25-40, 1978.

55. Chang L.W. Neurotoxic effects of mercury - A review. Environ Res. 14:329-373, 1977.

56. Clarkson T.W. The pharmacology of mercury compounds. Ann Rev Pharmacol. 12:375-406, 1972.

57. Stock A. Die Gefährlichkeit des Quecksilberdampfes und der Amalgame. Med. Klin. 22:1250-1252, 1926.

58. Schafer W.G., Hine M.K. and Levy B.M. A Textbook of Oral Pathology. W.B. Saunders Co, Philadelphia, 1974.

59. Ziff M.F. Mercury amalgam fillings and periodontal disease. Bio-Probe Newsletter 2(5):2-8, 1985.

60. Östlin L. et al. Amalgam Removal - A Road To Better Health? Health Insurance Bureau, Stockholm County Sweden, 1991.

61. Zamm AV. Removal of dental mercury: Often an effective treatment for the very sensitive patient. J Orthomol Med 5(3):138-142, 1990.

62. Ziff S and Ziff MF. Dental Mercury - An Environmental Hazard! Bio-Probe Newsletter 8(5):1-6, Sept 1992.

63. Nakayama H. et al. Mercury exanthem. Contact Dermatitis 9:411-417, 1983.

64. Arena J.M. Poisoning (4th ed.) Charles C. Thomas. Springfield, IL, 1979.

65. Gosselin R.E., Smith R.P. and Hodge H.C. Clinical Toxicology of Commercial Products. (95th ed). Williams and Wilkins, Baltimore, MD, 1984.

66. Leonhardt H. Fundamentals of Electro Acupuncture According to Voll. Haug CIE Nachf. BmBH, West Germany.

67. Vimy MJ and Lorscheider FL Intra-oral air mercury released from dental amalgam. J Dent Res 64:1069-1071, 1985.

68. Vimy MJ and Lorscheider FL. Serial measurements of intra-oral air mercury: Estimation of daily dose from dental amalgam. J Dent Res 64:1072-1075, 1985.

69. Vimy M.J., Luft A.J. and Lorscheider F.L. Estimation of mercury body burden from dental amalgam: Computer simulation of a metabolic compartmental model. J Dent Res 65(12):1415-1419, Dec 1986.

70. Cherian M.G. et al. Radioactive mercury distribution in biological fluids and excretion in human subjects after inhalation of mercury vapor. Arch Environ Health. 33(3):109-114, 1978.

71. Eggleston D.W. Effect of dental amalgam and nickel alloy on T-lymphocytes: Preliminary report. J Prosthet Dent. 51(5):617-623, 1984.

72. Shapiro IM; Berthold P; Mayro J; Vitale L; Rooney C; and Shenker BJ. Effects of mercuric compounds on human lymphocytes and monocytes. J Dent Res 71 (IADR Abstracts) 1992. Page 624, Abstract 874.

73. Shenker BJ; Rooney C; Vitale L; and Shapiro LM. Suppression of Human T and B cell activation by mercuric compounds. J Dent Res 71 (IADR Abstracts) 1992. Page 625, Abstract 875.

74. Smith D.C. and Williams D.F. Biocompatibility of Dental Materials, Vol III: Biocompatibility of Dental Restorative Materials. CRC Press, Inc., Boca Raton, FL 1982.

75. Wyman R.J. The Posterior Composite Resin Restoration. Winning at Restorative Dentistry Without Mercury. Maxplax, Toronto, Canada. 1984.

76. Clifford WJ. Materials Reactivity Testing - Background, basis and procedures for the immunological evaluation of systemic sensitization to components which emanate from biomaterials. (1990) Available from Clifford Consulting & Research, P.O. Box 17597, Colorado springs, CO 80935. (719) 599-8883.

77. Maryniuk G.A. In search of treatment longevity - A 30 year perspective. JADA 109(5):739-744, 1984.

78. Walls AWG, Wallwork MA, Holland IS, and Murray JJ. The longevity of occlusal amalgam restorations in first permanent molars of child patients. Br. Dent J. 158:133-136, 1985.

79. Clean Up. The new plastic aspirating device is available through Future Dentistry, P.O. Box 608634, Orlando, FL 32860-8634. Telephone (800) 282-9670.

80. Rom W.N. (Ed) In: Environmental and Occupational Medicine, page 461, Little, Brown and Co., Boston. 1983.

81. Dilley, D.H. et al. Time required for placement of alloy versus resin posterior restorations. Abstract #1583, page 340, J Dent Res 65, 1985.

82. ADA Letter dated February 19, 1985 signed by J.M. Coady, D.D.S., Executive Director.

83. Klassen CD, Amdur MO, Doull J. (Ed's) In: Casarett and Doull's Toxicology The Basic Science of Poisons (3rd Ed) page 606. Macmillan Publishing Co. 1986.

84. ADA News. Vol 16, Number 21, Nov 4, 1985.

APPENDIX A
PRE- AND POST-AMALGAM REPLACEMENT TESTING
TO ESTABLISH ACCEPTABLE DOCUMENTATION OF MERCURY BODY BURDEN RELATED TO THE PRESENCE OF AMALGAM DENTAL FILLINGS

Usually the immediate and primary goal of anyone who has been sick for any length of time is to just get better. Psychologically, the long suffering person is usually not interested in documenting the cause of their illness but rather only the "cure." It is not until after recovery from their health problems that they begin to dwell on the cause of their illness. Failure to take the time to document the cause of their previous illness or health condition frequently results in difficulty in obtaining insurance coverage for the procedures performed.

As a direct result of the many letters and conversations we have had with individual patients and dentists about this particular aspect of their treatment and recovery, we have elected to include a brief outline of the various tests that can be done to help document whether or not the amalgam dental fillings were in fact causally related to any health problems experienced.

The first criteria, of course, is that testing must be done prior to amalgam replacement and implementation of any detoxification protocols. This is necessary to establish a "base line" of values. Once a base line has been established for all the values to be monitored, then these values can be monitored by subsequent testing to determine whether changes that occur in the individual's health and base line values have any relationship to the elimination of mercury-containing dental fillings. Unfortunately, unless prescribed by a physician, most of the testing protocols we will describe will have to be paid for by the individual. These are all expenses that will be over and above those related to your dental treatment plan. However, they may serve as the basis for medical/dental insurance coverage and reimbursement by your insurance carrier.

ESTABLISHING YOUR INDIVIDUAL BASE LINE VALUES

1. Hair Analysis. This is a simple test that has been around for many years. However, it was not until recently that sufficient published research studies have clearly documented the validity of hair analysis for heavy metal screening. Although human hair primarily reflects organic mercury, studies have indicated that from 10-20% is inorganic mercury.(1) Regardless of composition, high mercury hair values, without any external source of exposure should be a matter of concern. A recent EPA report indicates that human hair is excellent for biological monitoring of mercury.(2)

2. Urine mercury, lead, copper, tin, and albumin. (The reason for taking lead levels is two-fold: 1) to rule out lead toxicity, or to show that the toxic effects of mercury are increased when lead is present. 2) Lead inhibits the enzyme delta-aminolevulinic acid dehydratase (ALA-D) and causes an increased excretion of delta-aminolevulinic acid (ALA). Mercury inhibits delta-aminolevulinic acid dehydrogenase, also identified as ALA-D.(3) If lead is not a factor but urine ALA-D is increased, then blood levels of ALA-D should be checked to see if either enzyme, dehydratase or dehydrogenase, has been inhibited, which would further tend to support the toxicity of the mercury body burden.

Copper, silver and tin are also given off by amalgam fillings. The presence of high copper, silver or tin in the urine could further indict amalgam fillings. Urine albumin may be indicative of mercury burden. The excretion of albumin is decreased during acute or chronic exposure to mercury. Research has shown an increase or normalization of urine albumin after replacement of amalgam fillings.

3. Urine mercury porphyrin profile. The testing of porphyrins is not new; what is new is that Dr. James Woods and his colleagues at the University of Washington at Seattle have refined the High Performance Liquid

Chromatograph (HPLC) technique for the testing of porphyrins that can produce a profile specific to mercury.(4) In the near future, major diagnostic testing laboratories should be able to perform the special HLPC porphyrin profile.

4. Fecal metal screen. This is a single-sample, one-pass analysis of a stool specimen that provides information on 25 different elements. This is a major route of excretion for mercury and silver, yet it is a valid test that is seldom, if ever, performed to check for heavy metal body burden. Production and collection of this type of data would permit establishing correlations between the health condition of an individual, the numbers and surfaces of amalgam dental fillings and fecal content of mercury as well as other amalgam metals such as silver, copper, tin and zinc.(5)

As explained in Appendix B, fecal analysis also presents a method of tracking and documenting an individuals progress towards better health. We have been unsuccessful in locating a certified laboratory in the U.S. with the necessary equipment, or the willingness to do commercial fecal metal screens of multiple metals. One reason for this may be the tremendous cost and effort involved. For example, we have been advised that the instrumentation itself costs over five million dollars and that calibration of the instrument for validity of results, can take two to three years. We consider the use of this type of analysis so important to the mercury intoxicated individual that we have established a working relationship with the laboratory in Sweden doing this type of analysis. The service will be made available through your dentist or physician. Anyone interested in securing a fecal analysis please have your dentist or physician contact Bio-Probe at (800) 282-9670 for more information.

5. Intra-oral mercury vapor levels, before stimulation by chewing gum for 10 minutes and after chewing gum for 10 minutes. The approved IAOMT intra-oral protocol should be utilized. This test is not diagnostic of mercury intoxication. It will, however, provide an evaluation of

how much mercury is being released from your amalgam dental fillings. The significance of this information is that science has clearly demonstrated that 80 to 100% of inhaled mercury vapor is absorbed from the lungs into the blood stream where it is then distributed throughout the body. From a documentation standpoint, intra-oral mercury vapor readings pre-amalgam removal and post-amalgam removal will clearly demonstrate your exposure to mercury vapor from your amalgam dental fillings.

6. Blood mercury levels. Whenever possible, any other blood base-lines desired should be done at the same time blood samples are taken to determine blood mercury levels. Although blood mercury levels are not diagnostic of chronic mercury toxicity, there is published research showing a decline in blood mercury levels after elimination of mercury-containing dental fillings.

7. Saliva mercury, copper and tin levels. "No mercury has been detected in saliva samples unless there was a mercury vapor exposure. Salivary glands are primary organs of excretion of mercury, and excessive exposure to inorganic mercury can result in salivary gland enlargement as well as excessive salivation....Salivary mercury levels can be much higher than blood mercury levels...."(6)

8. MetaMetrix, Inc. has developed a test to determine functional liver detoxication capacity. Based on a caffeine challenge, saliva is evaluated for the disappearance of caffeine, which has been determined to be a direct indicator of cytochrome P-450 activity.(7) Because there is documented scientific information showing the inhibition of cytochrome P-450 by mercury, this particular test or other possible tests for cytochrome P-450 could be of major medical import in establishing what role, if any, mercury from mercury dental implants plays in the ability of the liver to detoxify xenobiotics.(8) In this regard, if post-replacement testing is done, it would confirm a change in cytochrome P-450 activity based solely on removing a chronic mercury exposure source.

9. Current scientific research is demonstrating that cysteine and glutathione status have a very definite influence on efficiency of immune function.(9,10) It could be of extreme significance to show a variation in blood and/or urine sulfur amino levels pre and post amalgam replacement.

MERCURY CHALLENGE OR MOBILIZATION TESTING.

After establishing a urine mercury base-line. It is extremely important to then subject the patient to a test that would have a bearing on demonstrating body burden. At the present time, science has established that approximately 80% of the mercury body burden is contained in the kidneys. The other 20% being distributed to the brain, other organs and glands. The express purpose of a challenge test, is to administer a chelating agent, that has been scientifically documented to bind mercury and cause its excretion from the body. Several are available. At the present time there are three FDA approved drugs that can be used for this purpose: 1) British Anti-Lewisite (BAL), which is dimercaprol. Although effective and in use for more than 70 years, it does have many disagreeable and serious side-effects; 2) Penicillamine has also been used by the medical profession for a great number of years and it too has many side-effects; 3) 2-3 Dimercaprol succinic acid (DMSA) is the newest drug. It is a water soluble derivative of BAL that was approved by the FDA, in March of 1991, as a product to remove lead from children. However, it is also very effective for mercury and has minimal side effects.

The following protocol for DMSA has been derived from the published literature and the Physicians' Desk Reference: Provide the patient with a prescription to purchase DMSA. Quantity of 100 mg capsules is determined by using 30 mg/kg of patient body weight, i.e., a 150 lb individual

1 (75 kg) would require 75 x 30 = 2250 mg or 23 (100 mg) capsules. Provide the patient with a 24 hour urine collection kit and instructions for standard collection procedures (provided by the laboratory you intend to have do the analysis).

The DMSA is to be taken in three divided doses, 6 hours apart. All drugs, vitamins, minerals, amino acids should have been stopped for 24 hours prior to taking the DMSA and no supplements or drugs should be taken during the 24 hour period of urine collection. The decision regarding stopping any prescription medication for 48 hours to accomplish the Mobilization Test can only be done with written concurrence of a physician. Care must be taken not to contaminate the collection container. Starting at 6:00 A.M. take the first dose of DMSA. Collect the first urine starting at 8:00 A.M., and the patient must collect all urine voided for the next 24 hours. Take the 2nd dose of DMSA at noon and the 3rd dose at 6:00 P.M. Continue urine collection until 8:00 A.M. the following morning. Medication and any supplementation may begin again after completion of urine collection.

A mobilization blood sample should also be taken. The blood sample should be taken anytime between two and four hours after ingesting the first dose of DMSA (8:00 A.M.-10:00 A.M.). Samples should be assayed for mercury utilizing the same facility and procedure utilized to establish base-line blood mercury levels.

REFERENCES

1. Katz SA and Katz RB. Use of hair analysis for evaluating mercury intoxication of the human body: a review. J App Toxicol. 12(2):79-84, 1992.
2. Jenkins DW. Biological Monitoring of Toxic Trace Metals. Volume 1. Biological Monitoring and Surveillance. EPA-600/3-80-89. Pages 163-164, September 1980.
3. Homburger F; Hayes JA; Pelikan EW, Editors. A Guide To General Toxicology. Pages 233-235. Karger Continuing Education Series, Vol. 5. S. Karger AG, Switzerland. 1983.
4. Woods J. et al. Quantitative Determination of Porphyrins in Rat and Human Urine and Evaluation of Urinary Porphyrin Profiles During Mercury and Lead Exposures. Lab Clin Med, 129(2):272-281, Aug 1992.

5. Skare I and Engqvist A. Amalgam restorations - an important source to human exposure of mercury and silver. LÄKARTIDNIGEN 15:1299-1301, 1992. (English translation by authors available through Bio-Probe).

6. Stoppford, W. Chapter 15, Industrial exposure to mercury, page 387, in The Biogeochemistry of Mercury in the Environment, J.O. Nriagu Editor. Elsevier/North-Holland Biomedical Press, New York, 1979.

7. Functional Liver Detoxication Capacity Analysis. MetaMetrix, Inc. Medical Laboratory. 5000 Peachtree Industrial Blvd., Suite 110, Norcross, Georgia 30071. J. Alexander Bralley, Ph.D. Laboratory Director. (404) 446-5483. FAX (404) 441-2237. Also see "Metabolic Detoxification and Managing the Chronically Ill Patient" by Jeffery Bland, Ph.D. HealthComm, Inc. P.O. Box 1729, Gig Harbor, WA 98335. (206) 851-3943 or (800) 843-9660.

8. Veltman JC. and Maines MD. Alterations of Heme, Cytochrome P-450, and Steroid Metabolism by Mercury in Rat Adrenal. Archives Biochem Biophys. 248 (2):467-478, 1986.

9. DeFlora S. et al. antioxidant activity and other mechanisms of thiols involved in chemoprevention of mutation and cancer. The Am J Med. 91(suppl 3C):122S-130S, Sept 30, 1991.

10. Eck HP et al. Low concentrations of acid-soluble thiol (cysteine) in the blood plasma of HIV-1 infected patients. Biol Chem Hoppe Seyler 370:101-108, 1989.

63

INFORMED CONSENT

I _____ give my dentist _____ permission to remove servicable dental amalgam fillings and other nonprecious metals from my teeth and replace them with dental materials considered to be biocompatibile based on existing scientific research. These materials may include, but are not limited to, composite resins, ceramic, porcelain, gold alloys and titanium.

My dentist has provided me with a personal copy of the book *Dentistry Without Mercury*, which explains the pros and cons on the use of amalgam as a dental material and also gives the position of the American Dental Association on the safety of dental amalgam. Any questions I had that were not answered by this book were subsequently answered to my satisfaction by my dentist.

My dentist has explained to me that:

1. Although one or more of my subjective or objective signs or symptoms may resemble the signs or symptoms of mercury toxicity, I understand that this does not mean that I am suffering from the effects of mercury toxicity either directly or indirectly.

2. There is no scientific evidence that removal of my amalgam dental fillings will cure or improve any signs, symptoms, problems or health conditions that I have.

3. Any sign, symptom, problem or health condition that I have outside the mouth may involve a general health or medical question. My dentist is limiting advice to the mouth, and recommends that I consult a physician for any general health or medical concerns or questions which I have. Further, my dentist has not told me or represented to me that replacing my amalgam fillings or nonprecious metals would have any beneficial health effect on me at all.

If a posterior composite resin is the material chosen to replace dental amalgam and other nonprecious materials, the advantages and disadvantages of the material chosen have been explained to me, including the fact that there has not been a sufficient number of years of use to scientifically prove its wear characteristics. Accordingly, at this time, it is not known if posterior composites will last as long as dental amalgam and therefore may have to be replaced more frequently than amalgam. The pros and cons of other available alternative dental materials has also been explained to me.

As might occur with the placement of amalgam, gold, or any other dental material, I understand that there are situations beyond the control of my dentist that may necessitate endodontic treatment or removal of an existing tooth despite precautions taken and proper procedures utilized. In addition, I understand that during the removal and replacement of dental materials, it is possible to have an allergic type reaction to products used that may require immediate treatment. There is also a more delayed allergic reaction which is like a general sickness. Should I begin feeling poorly for no explained reason, I understand that it is my responsibility to advise my dentist immediately and to seek medical treatment.

My questions concerning the treatment plan recommended by my dentist and agreed to by me have been fully answered and I have read this statement and am satisfied that I have been fully informed.

Signature: _____ Date: _____

Please Print Name: _____

Witness: _____ Date: _____

Please Print Name _____

MEDICAL HISTORY

Date and purpose of most recent medical examination: _____

Name of physician: _____ phone: _____

Are you presently under medical care? _____ Reason: _____

Medications you are now taking: _____

WOMEN: Are you pregnant? _____ Month: _____ Nursing _____

Have you ever had radiation treatment for cancer? _____

Vitamin/Mineral supplements you are now taking: _____

Allergies: Medications: _____

Other Allergies: _____

Please check any of the following which you had or have been treated for:

___ Heart attack	___ Gum Disease/Bleeding	___ Irritability
___ Heart murmur	___ Periodontal disease (Pyorrhea)	___ Nervousness
___ Other heart disease	___ Mouth Ulcers	___ Anxiety
___ Heart Surgery/Pacemaker	___ Foul Breath	___ Depression
___ Angina/Chest pain	___ TMJ Syndrome/pain	___ Apathy
___ Irregular Heartbeat	___ Increased Salivation	___ Inability to concentrate
___ Tachycardia (racing heartbeat)	___ Metallic taste	___ Loss of memory
___ Rheumatic fever	___ Burning sensation in mouth	___ Fits of Anger
___ Stroke	___ Tremor (trembling)	___ Insomnia

_____ Cancer
_____ Bleeding problem
_____ Circulatory problem
_____ Anemia
_____ High Blood Pressure
_____ Low blood pressure
_____ Diabetes
_____ Hypoglycemia
_____ Arthritis
_____ Ulcers
_____ Kidney infection/failure
_____ Hepatitis/jaundice
_____ Hypo/Hyper thyroid
_____ Tuberculosis
_____ Emphysema
_____ Adrenal disease
_____ Venereal disease
_____ Epilepsy/seizures/convulsions
_____ Psychiatric treatment

_____ Numbness/Tingling sensations
_____ Joint pains
_____ Leg cramps
_____ Ringing noises in ears
_____ Chronic Headaches
_____ Neck/Spine problems
_____ Chronic Fatigue
_____ Low body temperature
_____ Skin rash
_____ Acne
_____ Nausea/vomiting
_____ Edema
_____ Restricted/dim vision
_____ Sensitivity to light
_____ Speech Disorders
_____ Abdominal cramps
_____ Colitis/diverticulitis
_____ Frequent constipation
_____ Persistent Diarrhea

_____ Suicidal tendencies
_____ Anorexia (poor appetite)
_____ Cold hands & feet
_____ Frequent urination
_____ Excessive perspiration
_____ Swollen lymph nodes
_____ Breathing difficulty
_____ Persistent cough
_____ Chronic sinus congestion
_____ Hay fever/Asthma
_____ Glaucoma
_____ Shingles
_____ Bell's Palsy
_____ PMS
_____ Multiple Sclerosis
_____ Lupus erythematosus
_____ Leukemia
_____ Hodgkin's Disease

Other serious illnesses or major surgery _____

Signature (Patient/Parent/Guardian): _____ Date: _____

DIRECTORY OF ORGANIZATIONS

- Foundation For Toxic Free Dentistry
  P.O. Box 608010, Orlando, FL 32860-8010   (1)
- International Academy of Oral Medicine and Toxicology
  P.O. Box 608531, Orlando, FL 32860-8531   (1) (2)
- American College of Advancement in Medicine
  23121 Verbugo Dr., Suite 204; Laguna Hills, CA 92653
  714-583-7666   (3)
- American Academy of Biological Dentistry
  P.O. Box 856; Carmel Valley, CA 93924   (1)
- Association of Health Practitioners.
  P.O. Box 5007, Durango, CO 81301   (1) (2)
- Queen and Company Health Communications, Inc.
  P.O. Box 49308; Colorado Springs, CO 80819-9938   (1) (2)
- National Center for Homeopathy
  1500 Massachusetts Ave. N.W.; Washington D.C. 20005   (1) (2)
- International Academy of Nutrition and Preventive Medicine
  P.O. Box 18433, Asheville, NC 28814   (1) (2)
- American Academy of Environmental Medicine
  P.O. Box 16016; Denver, CO 80216   (2)
- American Holistic Medical Association
   4101 Lake Boone Trail, Suire 201, Raleigh, NC 27607-6518   (2)(3)
- Dr. Jerry Mittelman
  263 West End Ave., #2A; New York, NY 10023   (1)
- Environmental Dental Association;
  9974 Scripps Ranch Blvd., Suite #36, San Diego, CA 92131   (1) (2)
- Huggins Diagnostic Center.
  5080 List Dr.; Colorado Springs, CO 80919   (1) (2)
- Roy Kupsinel, M.D.
  P.O. Box 550; Oviedo, FL 32765   (2)

(1) May be able to provide the name of a dentist in your area
who is familiar with the mercury amalgam toxicity issue and
the correct protocols for replacement.

(2) May be able to provide the name of a physician in your area
who is knowledgeable about mercury and other toxic metals.

(3) May be able to provide the name of a physician in your area
who has certified skills in detoxification therapy.

FOUNDATION FOR TOXIC FREE DENTISTRY

The Foundation For Toxic Free Dentistry has been established to fulfill several vital functions:

1. To gather accurate information on the health effects of materials used in dental treatment.

2. To distribute this information to its membership by means of a newsletter.

3. To assist in the distribution of this information to the general public.

4. To provide assistance in the legal defense of the right of the public to receive this information and the right of professionals to provide this information and allied services to their patients.

5. To gather and disseminate information on nutrition and diet in relation to oral health and disease.

6. To provide referrals to dentists (physicians whenever possible) familiar with the literature on mercury toxicity and who realize that amalgam dental fillings provide the greatest source of chronic exposure to mercury vapor and abraded amalgam particles.

The Foundation has been established as a not-for-profit organization, similar to a highly successful and influential group that has been in operation for a number of years in Sweden.

The Swedish group was organized to provide a support organization for those individuals who felt that they had been poisoned by their mercury amalgam dental fillings. This organization has been very effective in bringing the potential toxicity of mercury amalgam fillings to the attention of the Swedish media, public and the Swedish Parliament. The Foundation hopes to be just as effective in this country.

A number of potentially harmful materials are routinely used in the course of dental treatment. Dental materials that have been known to present possible health risks include: Mercury; nickel; beryllium; chrome; cobalt; copper; silver; and radioactive uranium.

The use of these materials presents a unique threat in that they are routinely placed directly in the body, often for long periods of time. Furthermore, the environment in which they are placed, the oral cavity, is uniquely harsh and suitable for transfer of these materials into the body cells themselves.

A determined minority of scientists and professionals has focused attention on evidence that these materials may present significant health risks to patients. Worldwide, more and more research is appearing that casts significant doubt on the wisdom of using these materials for dental treatment.

There is more than sufficient evidence casting doubt on the safety of the mercury released from dental amalgam fillings to constitute a legitimate scientific issue. This fact notwithstanding, the American Dental Association is busy reaffirming the safety of dental amalgam. In fact, the entire dental establishment seems to be mobilizing their efforts and resources to brand as quackery or fraud any statements or actions contrary to their established policy of saying that it is perfectly safe to implant a poison in your body, except in those few rare instances when the individual may be allergic to the poison.

Do you have the right to know what materials are placed in your mouth? Do you have the right to know what possible effect they may have on your health or that of your children? Are you aware that the causes of many common disease states are not known by the medical profession? Did you know that exposure to heavy metals, particularly mercury vapor, can cause pathological damage that is indicative of many of these disease states?

Evidently, the American Dental Association does not believe that you have any of the rights outlined above because in June of 1987 they took the unprecedented

70

action of inserting into their Principles of Ethics and Code of Professional Conduct, Section 1-J, a provision making it improper and unethical to remove amalgam restorations from the non-allergic patient for the alleged purpose of removing toxic substances from the body, when such treatment is performed solely at the recommendation or suggestion of the dentist. In effect, this limits your dentist from even mentioning the potential hazards of the mercury being constantly released from any silver mercury fillings that you may have.

It is the Foundation's position that this is a clear violation of the rights of both the patient and the doctor and a misguided attempt to suppress scientific and medical progress. There is an effort underway in some states to enact legislation that will permit physicians and dentists to practice alternative therapies and to also insure that the patient's right to information is not arbitrarily limited by special interest groups.

PATIENT ADVERSE REACTION REPORT.(PARR)

FTFD has developed a two part form that is being used to report information to the U.S. Food and Drug Administration (FDA). Each patient who is having or has had their mercury-containing dental fillings replaced with non-mercury dental fillings should complete a PARR form. In your own words, the patient lists the major health problems or symptoms that existed prior to having their amalgam dental fillings exchanged for non-mercury containing fillings. Approximately six-months after the last filling has been replaced, the patient indicates on the form following the original health problem whether their condition improved, remained the same, or got worse. The original of the PARR form is sent to the FDA and the duplicate copy is forwarded to the FTFD. The FTFD has established a computer file for each form and every symptom or problem listed is entered along with the results of amalgam replacement. Statistics such as those displayed on page 41 are derived from the file. The FDA has also established a computer file on the PARR forms submitted

71

to them. Anyone desiring a PARR form can have one by requesting it from FTFD.

DENTAL & HEALTH FACTS

The Foundation Newsletter "Dental & Health Facts" will provide supporters and the general public the latest information on dental materials and new techniques and procedures for their use. It will also provide nutritional information related to the oral environment considered to be of interest and concern to the members. Perhaps more importantly, it will on a national basis attempt to keep the membership abreast of all the legal and legislative information related to the basic issues.

One other major service the Foundation provides is referrals to mercury-free dentists. These are dentists who have indicated that they do not place mercury/amalgam dental fillings any longer. Moreover, these dentists have a true appreciation for the great amount of mercury vapor that can be generated during removal operations and use every precaution available to protect and minimize unnecessary patient and staff exposures. They should all have training and have extensive experience in the proper placement of alternative composite materials. Having said all that, the reader must understand that neither the Foundation, nor the DAMS coordinators have personal knowledge of most of the dentists on their referral lists. Consequently, you must call and by asking intelligent questions determine if the dentist you have been referred to is acceptable to you. The first question of course is "Do you place amalgam fillings?" If the answer is yes, look for another dentist. If the answer is NO then you should be concerned with how long they have been mercury-free and their experience and training in the placement of composites.

For a free sample issue of the Foundation Newsletter, PARR form, or referral to the closest mercury-free dentist they have on their list, simply send your request to FTFD or FOUNDATION FOR TOXIC FREE DENTISTRY, P.O.

72

BOX 608010, ORLANDO, FL 32860-8010. Please also include with your request a #10 self addressed and stamped envelope.

If you wish to join the Foundation, include a check or money order payable to FTFD or Foundation For Toxic Free Dentistry in the amount of $15.00 in U.S. funds. Membership applications from foreign countries (other than Canada) please add an additional $15.00 to cover the increased postage costs (total $30.00 U.S.).

The FTFD is staffed by all volunteer help and all monies collected are used only for approved FTFD projects. Additional contributions are welcomed. The Foundation For Toxic Free Dentistry is a 501(c)(3) nonprofit tax-exempt organization. Your gifts are tax deductible to the full extent the law allows.

DENTAL AMALGAM MERCURY SYNDROME
(DAMS)

Some very wonderful people, most of them prior victims of mercury poisoning from their mercury/amalgam dental fillings, have started forming victim support groups, most bearing the name DAMS. These individuals feel a strong obligation to their fellow citizens to inform them of the potential health hazards of inhaling mercury vapor and swallowing abraded particles of mercury from their amalgam dental fillings 24 hours a day, 365 days a year.

Although removal of mercury/amalgam dental fillings does not guarantee health improvements, most people who have replaced their mercury fillings with gold or composite fillings have experienced reversal or improvement of persistent health problems. Many experienced these life-altering improvements after years of suffering and frustration without ever receiving a valid medical diagnosis or having the cause of their health problem identified. the symptom (See symptom analysis on Page 31)

That unfortunate situation stems from the fact that most physicians have been lulled, by the dental establishment, into believing that mercury released from amalgam dental fillings poses no threat to health except in those few people who may be allergic to it. Consequently, most physicians have never previously taken the patient very seriously when they asked "Can the mercury from my dental fillings be causing my health problems?" Science and clinical case histories are beginning to change that attitude.

There is a grass-roots movement across this country to require that every dental patient be given their constitutional right to FREEDOM OF CHOICE to say NO to mercury amalgam dental fillings for themselves and their loved ones; to promote the public's RIGHT TO KNOW the potential health hazards of constant daily exposure to mercury from mercury dental fillings and to insure that concerned dentists have the right to inform their patients of this issue.

The dedicated individuals involved in the DAMS groups are all victims and all volunteers. They are trying to provide understanding and information to those individuals bewildered by their health conditions, and who are trying to gain additional knowledge about the potential health effects of mercury. DAMS coordinators may also be able to refer you to a mercury-free dentist in your area. It is important that you extend these people the courtesy of only writing to them initially if you are soliciting any information or help. There just aren't enough hours in the day for them to talk to everyone by telephone.

There are now over 60 different support groups around the country. As more and more people become active on the issue, new DAMS units are being formed almost every month. Consequently, we can only provide a partial list of some of the DAMS organizations.

Murlene Brake, DAMS of New Mexico. 725-9 Tramway Lane, NE, Albuquerque, NM 87122 publishes a National DAMS Newsletter. The subscription price is $15.00 per year. Murlene keeps a master list of all the DAMS organizations in the country. You can write her for any DAMS organizations in your state.

Louise Herbeck, DAMS of Illinois. P.O. Box 9065, Downers Grove, IL 60515. Louise is one of the co-founders of DAMS in the United States. Louise has also appeared on several TV talk shows, was on the 60 Minute program December 16, 1990 "Is Their A Poison In Your Mouth" and has made many presentations in the Chicago area.

Shirley Brown, DAMS of Colorado. P.O. Box 19032, Denver, CO 80209 also publishes a Newsletter. Shirley is the other co-founder of DAMS and has been very active in the organization. Shirley has appeared on TV and radio talk shows, letting people know about the issue and that there is help for those who need it. Subscriptions to her Newsletter are also $15.00 per year.

Carolyn Smith, DAMS of Michigan, 426 Grant, Grand Haven, MI 49417. Has been very active in Michigan and has had several articles published in various Newspapers.

Robert O. Stephenson, DAMS of Alaska. 1837 No Way Lane, Fairbanks, AK 99079-6338. Bob has done an outstanding job in the state of Alaska and has been instrumental in insuring that various government agencies are aware of potential health hazards of amalgam fillings.

Cheryl Quackenbush, ADAMS, P.O. Box 854, Kirkland, WA 98083-0854. Cheryl and her group have been very active in the State of Washington and have been instrumental in having proposed unfavorable administrative rulings on the amalgam issue withdrawn..

Our special thanks to all the other DAMS coordinators doing wonderful things in their own states.

FTFD MEMBERSHIP APPLICATION

Yes: I want to support the Foundation for Toxic Free Dentistry and the legal challenge to my constitutional rights to be told about the dangers of mercury or other dental materials. I understand that as a member I will receive the Foundation's Dental & Health Facts Newsletter.

Name _____

Address _____

City _____

State/Zip _____

Signature _____

The Foundation For Toxic Free Dentistry is a 501(c)(3) non-profit tax-exempt organization. Your gift is tax deductible to the full extent the law allows

ANNUAL RATES/INFORMATION		
	Category	Amount
☐	Membership Renewal	$15.00
☐	New Membership	$15.00
☐	Additional Donation	$_____
☐	Send Adverse Reaction Report	
☐	Refer me to a mercury-free dentist	

(RD93)